# SICK DOCTORS

# SICK DOCTORS

Edited by

## RAYMOND GREENE

WILLIAM HEINEMANN MEDICAL BOOKS LTD

First Published 1971.


© William Heinemann Medical Books Ltd 1971


ISBN 0 433 12602 7


Printed by photo-lithography and made in Great Britain at
the Pitman Press, Bath

# Preface

During a recent illness it became clear to me that the descriptions of the symptoms in medical "literature" were very inadequate. If this were true of my illness it seemed likely to be true of others. The explanation was obvious. The descriptions were "hearsay" only, second hand or worse.

In this book the symptoms of diseases are described at first hand by medical patients. If it serves a useful purpose it could be the first of a series. I hope that other sick doctors will be inspired to send me the stories of their illness.

R.G.

# Acknowledgements

The Editor wishes to acknowledge the following sources
for permission to reproduce copyright material.

*Chapter 3*   Reproduced by kind permission of the author.
Copyright © 1952, by The Atlantic Monthly
Company Boston, Mass. Reprinted with permission.

*Chapter 6*   Reproduced by kind permission of the author and
the editor of the *Lancet* in which it appeared in the
issue of November 22nd 1961.

*Chapter 8*   Reproduced by kind permission of the author and
the editor of the *Lancet* in which it appeared in the
issue of January 25th 1964.

*Chapter 19*  Reproduced by kind permission of the author and
the editor of the *British Medical Journal* in which it
appeared in the issue of July 18th 1970.

*Chapter 22*  This chapter is reproduced by kind permission of the
author.

# Contents

# Chapter I

# Acute Abdomen

In a forenoon, while driving along a highway on my way to work, I first experienced a "gas pain" in my epigastric region. I say "gas pain" since it was exactly the type of pain I had felt before in other parts of my abdomen when gas was trapped in a segment of intestine. The pain in these instances was relieved as gas moved on or was evacuated. However, on this occasion the "gas pain" persisted and although I changed my position in my seat in various ways I could not change the pain. Finally, because I had a sensation of "bloating", I loosened my belt, hoping this would help — it did not. I had no nausea and did not vomit, but was uneasy because of the epigastric discomfort. This lasted one or two minutes and after I changed positions further, the pain suddenly disappeared. However, almost as fast as the pain disappeared in the epigastrium a sharp pain appeared in my right lower quadrant. This caused me to slide down in the seat and flex my thigh. I used my left foot to drive the car which fortunately, or unfortunately, was now stopped in traffic. My abdomen to palpation was bony hard in all quadrants but not tender at all except in one small area in the right lower quadrant. I knew I had either a ruptured ulcer or acute obstruction of the appendix with rupture, but finally settled for the first diagnosis. Although the pain was bad, I can't say it was intense or unbearable. However, I must say I did not move about after the right lower quadrant pain appeared. I held myself in one position — semi-flexed and slouched down in the seat. I saw no point in calling for help since there were cars stopped in traffic on all sides of me and, at best, I figured I was thirty minutes from the hospital. As it turned out this was correct. I made it to my hospital and I parked. I'm sure that if I had pulled off the road, flagged another driver, and waited for an ambulance, much time would have been lost. At any rate, I was able to drive with my left foot and arrived at the hospital with relatively little severe pain.

After I parked my car and thought of moving from my crouched position I realized that this was going to be very painful even before I experienced the pain. However, I had no alternative

1

but to get out of the car since there was no one about to call. As soon as I stood up I felt as if I was cut in two by a terrible lacerating pain across my lower abdomen. This caused me to fall forward in a crouched position and, in fact, I fell across the fender to the ground. In this position I felt better. I signalled to a passer-by to get me a wheelchair from the hospital and it seemed as if he was never coming back, although I'm sure it was only a few minutes before he reappeared. Moving to the wheelchair was painful and I assumed my posture of forward flexion at the hips. Up to this time, I must say, for whatever the reason the pain had not taken possession of me. I could make decisions and was in control. Shortly thereafter this changed. As I was wheeled into the emergency room and I climbed up to the examining table, it seemed as if everything let go — me included. The pain was agonizing, causing me to scream and demand Demerol. Whether this was because I was now in the arms of a hospital I don't know, but it seemed as if everything was much more painful as I entered the protection of the accident room.

Of course, thereafter, I was examined by physicians. Of interest at this point was the fact that for the first time when I sat up severe pain appeared in my right acromio-clavicular joint area. This was painful to the touch also. As I lay down this disappeared but my shoulder was still sore on pressure. The pain in the shoulder could be reproduced at will by sitting up and relieved by lying down, but for several days after operation my shoulder was still surprisingly very sore. As a matter of fact, to this day, years later, it is still sore. Exercise, such as tennis, may have something to do with this, although I had never had it before.

At any rate, after drugs I felt much better and I must say that it was not only the absence of pain that changed but my mentation was affected. I felt as if I were floating and my response to everything was indeed modified. I'm sure if I had been told that they were going to cut my head off I would have replied, "of course", (the effect of Demerol). I could move without pain; in fact, climbed onto the operating table without any discomfort. This to me has always been remarkable since I felt that such mechanical distortion should produce more discomfort in the circumstances. However, it did not.

After the operation I had little discomfort except in the wound, nose and shoulder. The latter still bothered me at rest and on movement. The nasal gastric tube was intolerable and I urged my surgeon to remove it as soon as possible. I had little abdominal discomfort postoperatively except when laughing or moving. There was sharp wound pain for a moment for several days at these times but little or no pain relief was necessary; in fact, the one shot of morphine that I received immediately post-operatively gave me such an odd sensation that I refused all further routine analgesics. Of interest after a few days post-operatively, when I was out of bed, my pulse rate was the slowest (48) it has ever been; I suppose from total relaxation. I had the usual profound postoperative fatigue.

There were very comical events associated with all this. I won't belabour the point but one series of items seems noteworthy. After I was admitted to the emergency room the first doctor who saw me was a friend of mine, an obstetrician. While I was in the X-ray department, under drugs, he popped in again. In the operating room, as I was being "prepped", he was there, but I also realized that the nurse who was doing the abdominal preparation was a woman who had worked in the delivery room. Finally, after operation, there were no beds in the general hospital other than on the obstetric floor and I was delivered to one of these. Just then again, my obstetrician friend reappeared. All I could think is that there must have been some error and exclaimed, "My God — they couldn't have made this mistake!!!"

# Chapter II

# Aphthous Ulcers

I get ulcers in the mouth. The technical name is recurrent aphthous ulceration (minor variety). They make me ill-tempered, and so far no effective treatment has been found, and I have not yet discovered how to prevent them from developing. I hope I will, for I try anything that is suggested which has a rational basis (and some remedies that haven't).

It is said that 30% of the population develop such ulcers. One would have thought, therefore, that more would be known about them, or that an effective treatment would be available.

The ulcers to which I am referring are not associated with herpes simplex, nor are they the serious ulcers which leave scars, nor are they associated with any other disorder. They are the simple tender mouth ulcers which seem to come out of the blue and for which no apparent cause can be found.

After twenty-five years of close observation of these ulcers I feel that I can express some doubts concerning the accepted theories on their causation (at least as far as my own ulcers are concerned).

A micro-organism has been suspected to be the causative agent (the transitional L form of an alpha haemolytic streptococcus). This is hard to dispute, but I doubt if this micro-organism is more than an opportunist invader, like the *Demodex folliculorum* in rosacea.

Early in 1970 my two daughters and I all had ulcers simultaneously. Perhaps this was co-incidence. Perhaps we were all invaded by the organism at the same time; or perhaps one of the factors involved is a foodstuff which we had all eaten. This seems most likely, but attempts at reviewing our diet of the preceding days were inconclusive, so I have been trying to eliminate suspect foodstuffs one by one.

I must seem illogical to my acquaintances. For months I avoided nuts, until I developed ulcers while on a nut-free diet, so I reasoned that nuts were not the sole precipitating food. Then I had a strawberry-free period, then tomatoes, and now am trying the effect of avoiding pineapple.

This would appear to be easy at first sight but pineapple pops up unsuspectedly in all sorts of foods. It is often in desserts, and sometimes given with a curry; but one has to be careful of punch, pineapple centres in chocolates, Chinese meals, and savouries stuck on the end of little sticks at cocktail parties. The incidence of ulceration seems to be reduced just now, but a long period of observation is necessary, for the ulcers may not appear for six or eight weeks.

Their arrival is heralded by a sudden awareness of an unduly sensitive patch in the mouth. It may be a small ulcer, though sometimes it is a mucosal nodule. The nodule is not much to the observer, but the subject is well aware of it, and may even catch it accidentally when eating. We are very aware of minor changes in our mouths and even a tiny chip off a tooth constantly annoys us, until we get used to it. The nodule may last for three or four days before maturing into the round or oval ulcer with its yellowish grey base, erythematous surroundings and slight local oedema. The ulcer is tender and painful for six or seven days but the pain goes before the healing takes place. I cannot tell from inspection alone which ulcer is painful and which has passed the painful stage. Moreover the pain fluctuates during the day, being at its worst on arising and about 4.30 p.m. After ten to fourteen days the ulcer heals.

Unfortunately within a week or so I often seem to develop more ulcers. In fact there seems to be a definite cycle, not necessarily of ulceration, but of lowered resistance to whatever causes the ulceration. At times the prodromal feelings are there, but no ulcer develops.

During the course of my investigations into this problem I have taken smears from my oral mucosa for study after Shorr or Papanicolaou staining. I lightly scrape the buccal surface with a wooden spatula. I have had to suspend the study at times when I am ulcer-prone because ulceration has developed at the site of the trauma produced by the spatula. At other periods I can scrape the same area several times a day with no hint of ulceration.

Similarly during the past ten years I have had occasional attacks of low back pain for which I have at times taken phenylbutazone with no untoward effects. Last year, however, I developed severe ulceration of the tongue and oral mucosa after a few days on the usual dosage of phenylbutazone. I believe that this is because my ingestion of the drug on this occasion, for the first time, coincided with a period at which I was ulcer-prone.

In theory topical local anaesthetic agents should help. I have found them to be worse than useless. They deaden the pain for a while but cause a loss of feedback information concerning the position of the tongue and cheeks, with a resulting difficulty in speaking as clearly as usual. My patients look at me a bit strangely and I feel that they are debating whether or not I have been drinking. The edges of the ulcers themselves seem to stand out from the deadened surface and feel wooden. They are more prone to further trauma when speaking and eating. This is a time when trauma should be avoided, so I no longer use preparations containing topical anaesthetics. The application of phenol and similar substances is advocated, but I find their effect too short-lived.

Corticosteroids are recommended by many authors. The use of agents which inhibit healing does not seem logical to me, but I have tried them, sometimes in desperation. A painful ulcer on the tip of one's tongue before a busy clinic which involves talking to patients, medical students and nurses, repeatedly traumatizing the tender area, leads to trying any remedy which promises relief. In theory the steroid should lessen the inflammatory reaction around the ulcer, possibly lessening some of the pain. I have tried both hydrocortisone and the betamethasone pellets recommended for aphthous ulceration. Neither gave much relief, and when taken prophylactically for several weeks both failed to prevent the next crop of ulcers from developing. I found these tablets hard to manage. One cannot hold a tablet in the mouth for long when seeing patients, especially if the ulcer is in an awkward place. Mealtimes are equally unsuitable, and in the evenings one is lucky to be able to keep the pellet in position without causing some domestic strife by speaking only briefly. In fact driving a car alone provides one of the few opportunities modern man has of allowing the pellet to dissolve in situ according to the manufacturer's instructions. Since I live close to my work, however, I have had to drive round the district waiting for the pellet to dissolve, not unlike the G.P. who wants to hear the end of the programme on his car radio before visiting his patient. However I wonder if the action attributed to the steroid is not achieved by its systemic effect; in which case I am tempted to swallow the tablet. A steroid is available in a base said to be specially formulated for adhesion to the ulcerated area. It is said to leave a protective film. Twenty minutes is the longest I can get it to stick in my mouth.

Antihistamines, which have a local anaesthetic action, make no difference to my ulcers. Topical tetracycline mouth washes are effective in the herpetiform type of mouth ulceration, but do nothing for me. Some of my patients, however, get fewer ulcers when they take long-term tetracycline. This may be due (as may its efficacy in acne) to some property other than its antibiotic one. Some of my female patients are ulcer-free when pregnant or when taking "the pill". So far my ulceration has not been serious enough for me to try oestrogen therapy!

Carbenoxolone is reported to be of considerable use in ulceration lower down the gastro-intestinal tract, but does not seem to be as effective for aphthous ulceration. I have not been able to give it as long a trial as I would like because it makes me feel sick.

Until a better treatment is found I rely on salicylates. Aspirin is used as a gargle after tonsillectomy, after which it is swallowed. I dissolve a soluble aspirin tablet in a ¼ tumbler of water and hold the solution in the mouth in contact with the ulcers for half a minute or so before swallowing it. This eases the pain of the ulcers without deadening the tongue or affecting the speech. The effect lasts for only half an hour, so I sometimes have to repeat the performance once or twice a session, between patients. A salicylate gel is sold which acts in a similar manner, but I do not find it as effective.

I hope one day to come across a substance which will prevent these ulcers from forming. I believe that it will act by increasing the keratinization of the oral mucosa, for my observations indicate that whatever the causes of aphthous ulceration, they act on the areas of poorest keratinization and at times when the defence mechanisms of the mouth are at their least efficient.

Chapter III

# Blindness

The doctor's office was on 59th Street, and as we came out on the sidewalk we could see that the green of Central Park was beginning to be tinged with faint brown under the hot blue sky of mid-July. We went to Rumpelmayer's for lunch and afterwards took a taxi to the hospital. Riding uptown, I can remember seeing a sign above a shoe store. The letters were large, black upon a white background, and surrounded by a scintillating halo. They spelled out the words "Thom McAn", and they were the last I was ever to read. The next day I was operated upon for retinal detachment. Despite the efforts of an able surgeon, the operation was a failure and since that day twelve years ago I have been totally blind.

When my world thus came tumbling down about my ears, I was forty years old, with a wife and two small sons, aged six and eight years. I had been engaged in the practice and teaching of internal medicine for fifteen years and had attained the rank of assistant professor of clinical medicine in a large metropolitan school. At the age of five, I had been found to be a high myope with astigmatism and ocular muscle imbalance. Like many myopes I was an avid reader with a retentive, photographic memory, but despite my visual handicap I was also able to participate in sports, such as baseball and football, to a limited extent. My myopia increased sharply during adolescence, and by the time I was twenty-two years of age had reached 12 diopters During succeeding years, likewise, the imbalance of my ocular muscles and my astigmatism gradually became worse. When I was thirty-two, I suffered a large retinal tear in the macula of my left eye. The consensus of my ophthalmological consultants was against surgical repair, and for the next seven years I lived and worked with slowly failing monocular vision.

There is no need here to recount the thoughts, the desperate dwindling hopes, the slow surrender to grim inevitable truth of one who watches the dark curtain slowly descend; nor does it seem fitting to transcribe that black despair which twists the heart when the silent severance from light is made complete.

These things, portrayed by abler pens than mine, seemed to me to lie too deep for plucking forth and must remain visible only to one all-seeing eye. Suffice it to say that the storm was somehow weathered through. The facts being squarely faced, it became necessary to take stock and to make a decision. The inventory showed among our assets some pearls of great price. Chief among these stood my wife, herself a physician and gifted with intelligence, optimism and energy. Without her loyalty, and her gay courageous heart, a dark way would have been darker indeed. Her ability to achieve a career for herself, while maintaining to the fullest the role of wife and mother, and giving encouragement, guidance and support to me in a hundred ways, represents in itself a most noteworthy accomplishment. Next in importance stood the encouragement and support of my friends and colleagues, and the co-operation of my associates and superiors in the medical school and hospital. Fortunate also was the happy accident of my training in a special field where the benefit of vision is more dispensable, or rather less indispensable, than in most.

With these considerations in mind, only one decision was possible: to pick up the pieces and to carry on. Through the co-operation and kindness of hospital and academic authorities, I have been able to concentrate my activities in the teaching hospital of our medical school. My work has continued to include private consultation practice, the direction of a special out-patient clinic and clinical teaching in the form of bedside conferences, ward rounds and clinical lectures. I visit patients in consultation in their homes or other hospitals, sit on various hospital committees, contribute occasional articles to the medical literature and present papers from time to time before local or national medical organizations. My office and hospital practice is carried on with the aid of an assistant.

For various reasons I have failed to utilize several facilities of advantage to the blind. Thus, I have not attempted to learn Braille. This doubtless is due in large part to intrinsic inertia (a euphemism for pure laziness); to the ineptitude of a middle-aged set of reflexes; to the fact that much of my reading material is of necessity technical and not available in Braille, and in large measure to the availability of other sources of cultural and recreational reading. The *Talking Books*, made possible through the combined efforts of a government project and the American Foundation for the Blind, have filled a great need with the wide variety of literature which they supply. Radio has its obvious niche and, along with periodicals and newspapers read to me by members of my family, helps to keep me abreast of current developments. Much of my spare time is of necessity devoted to the current medical literature and the preparation of lectures. In this I have enjoyed the services of a neighbour, a skilled reader, versed in medical literature, the widow of a distinguished colleague and friend.

Two other potential advantages have likewise not been realized. The availability of stenographic assistants and technical recording facilities has abetted my disinclination to learn a touch system of typewriting (doubtless another manifestation of intrinsic inertia). I have not acquired a seeing-eye dog largely because most of my time is spent indoors within the hospital and office. The problem of physical exercise has been solved in part by cross-country walking and calisthenics.

What of the practice of medicine without benefit of vision? The effectiveness of the properly integrated use of palpation, an attentive ear and a keen olfactory sense is indeed remarkable. The auditory impression of the length of stride and the level from which the spoken voice emanates give a useful estimate regarding the height of the patient. The quality of the voice tells me much about the personality and emotional tension. The quality imparted by swelling of the upper respiratory mucous membranes or by motor impairment of the laryngeal mechanism is often characteristic. I have been able correctly to suspect the presence of acromegaly and of myxedema from the quality of the patient's voice. The vocal quality imparted by tumours in the nasopharynx, or by uvular paralysis or weakness, is sometimes diagnostic — as is the stridor associated with recurrent laryngeal paralysis or with intrathoracic pressure exerted upon the trachea or bronchi.

The uses of palpation are manifold and obvious. The patient's general habitus, his state of nutrition and of muscular tone and development, the presence of atrophy, and conformation of the skull, the physiognomy, the texture of the skin can be ascertained by touch. Also, the character and distribution of the hair, exophthalmos, oedema, the presence of tumours, adenopathy, goitre, vascular pulsation, ascites, hernias, lesions of the nails, tremors, enlargement of abdominal viscera, all these things and many more, are readily revealed to the exploring hand of the sightless examiner.

Likewise, the value of olfactory impressions is not inconsiderable. The fresh alcoholic aroma which surrounds the diurnal drinker, or the stale smell of last night's drinking bout, may reveal much. The odours imparted by the excessive smoking of cigarettes, cigars and pipe tobacco, are all characteristic. I once astonished a patient after we had exchanged a few words of introduction, by remarking that all I knew of him at the moment was that he had lived in New York, probably Brooklyn, and that he was a heavy smoker of cigars. He pleaded guilty to both these soft impeachments. The answers of course lay in his characteristic accent and the equally characteristic odour of cigar tobacco which hung about him. The quality of a woman's perfume and cosmetics, or the lack of them, may be revealing. The characteristic odours of disease require but little comment. Uraemia, acetonaemia and sometimes intestinal obstruction, all impart a characteristic quality to the breath of the patient. Clinicians of an older generation, lacking the diagnostic refinements of today, were obliged to rely more upon their senses, and I have heard them describe the characteristic smell of typhoid fever, smallpox, and other infectious diseases. I cannot vouch for the accuracy of these observations from my own experience.

Diagnosis — absolute or tentative — and a plan for further study or treatment thus crystallize from correlation of several components. The fundamental importance of a carefully detailed history seems too obvious for comment. Yet despite the emphasis placed upon it in curricula, and the recent renaissance of interest in the personal relationship between patient and physician, this art remains largely undeveloped among medical students and young physicians. Hurry is a major fault in the procurement of a history in office and clinic practice. It is of prime importance that the patient be put at ease and made to feel that he has plenty of time to tell his story to a sympathetic listener. It is admittedly sometimes difficult to reconcile such an attitude with the inevitable pressures of the day's work; but once this relationship is established, impressions of great value regarding the fundamental origin of the patient's complaints can often be obtained.

A careful history having been extracted and digested, those parts of the physical examination which are dependent upon the examiner's vision, such as the patient's colour, the appearance of the skin, the ocular findings, the appearance of the teeth, mouth, tongue, throat, and so forth, are completed by my assistant and I then proceed with my own part of the examination. After properly correlating the information thus obtained, I am able with the aid of a rather highly visual imagination to form an impression of the patient and his diagnostic problem, which is usually, I think, pretty close to that which would be gained by a sighted physician. It may be understood that I am obliged to depend more than the average internist upon the services of special consultants — the dermatologist, the ophthalmologist, the otolaryngologist, the electrocardiographer and the fluoroscopist.

The personal relationship between the patient and the blind physician deserves some comment. I am sure that many persons who would otherwise have consulted me have not done so — doubtless because they hesitate to entrust themselves to one who cannot see, and some perhaps because of an understandable philistinic complex which leads to the avoidance of affliction. Most of the patients who come to see me know that I am blind, and I see to it that the few who do not know, are soon tactfully made aware of the truth. I have occasionally been amused by patients who were not yet aware of my visual handicap asking whether I would personally perform a recommended surgical operation. The situation once understood, there is very likely to develop a sympathetic relationship between the patient and myself which I think is often deeper and stronger than that which exists between the ordinary doctor and his patient. There often follows a relaxation of mental reservation and a letting down of emotional barriers, a freedom of communication which is of inestimable value in many instances both to the patient and to me. This is of particular advantage in the recognition and management of the numerous functional and emotional disturbances which form so large and important a part of the practice of internal medicine. I have often thought that blindness might actually be at times an advantage to the psychiatrist. There are, I believe, a few blind psychiatrists practising at this time; and while I have not had the privilege of discussing this point with any one of them, I trust that I may one day be able to do so.

Most of the teaching in which I engage consists of clinical lectures to undergraduates and graduate groups and bedside clinical conferences with small groups of undergraduate students. The preparation of lectures requires much time, usually two to three hours for each hour of teaching and calls for the memorizing of a detailed outline. The problem of adjusting lectures to the passage of time has been solved by the use of a repeater watch or a Braille-type watch. My bedside conferences are based largely on the Socratic method and, as they consist largely of "spot" teaching, do not permit detailed preparation beyond a preliminary review of the general problem presented by the patient.

Corollary to the current progress in technology and educational methods, many fields of training are now available to those among the blind who cannot rely upon the development of natural aptitudes in literature, music, or the other arts. Among these special fields are several professions, including theology, social service, teaching and the law. I am sometimes asked whether in my opinion a blind person could successfully complete the required courses in a modern medical school. I am sure that under present conditions this would be an impossibility. The Keeneys, in their interesting article reviewing blindness among practising physicians, have outlined the careers of a number of outstanding blind physicians of ancient and modern times. Notable among such physicians are the late Dr. Robert Babcock of Chicago and Dr. Moorhead of Dublin. However, with the exception of Babcock, all of the blind physicians with whose careers I am familiar suffered their loss of vision after completing their medical education. Babcock, who lost his vision in boyhood, completed his education while totally blind. His remarkable accomplishments are outstanding.

What are the uses of my adversity? These may be catalogued as of the body, the mind and the spirit. Chief among the physical advantages which have accrued to me I would place the development of my auditory sense. There is a widespread belief among the laity that the blind are likely to be endowed with a compensatory increase in acuteness of hearing. This is not true. There is, of course, no physiological reason why blindness should be followed by an increase in auditory acuity. From my own experience, however, I am convinced that largely as a result of necessity, the blind are able to develop to a high degree their latent or innate ability to interpret and orient the significance of sounds. One learns to do perforce what one must do. Life in the great world of sound has been described in a fascinating way by sightless writers more gifted than myself. A keen awareness of many of the details of the life which is going on around and about us is possible to those who know how to use their ears to interpret what they hear. Thus, as I sit dictating these lines in my bedroom on a quiet midsummer morning, I am aware of many things. From the kitchen I can hear and smell the pleasant preparations for lunch; in the upstairs sitting room I can hear the metallic snip of my mother's scissors as she mends the torn trousers of her oldest grandson; in the field behind the back hedge a carpenter is hammering away. A soft wet wind laden with the promise of rain gently stirs the elm trees in the front yard; the milkman's electric truck whirrs to a quiet stop in front of the house. I hear him dismount, and rattling his bottles, walk up the gravel drive toward the kitchen door; a family of robins quarrel noisily in the garden; overhead hangs a crow with raucous, irritated cries; across the street the neighbour's children scold their dachshund; and from the distant highway comes the muffled, interrupted roar of the mid-morning traffic's strain.

I have learned to distinguish the individual characteristics of voices and speech which permit me to identify most of my friends after only a few words have been spoken. Aided by occasional brief descriptions of scene and action, I am able quite readily to follow plays on the stage or screen from dialogue alone. One minor accomplishment has interested me a good deal. I am somehow able to detect the proximity of a wall when I get within two or three feet of it. The most obvious explanation lies in the variation of reflected sound. Yet I have on occasion been able to make such identification in the apparent absence of sources of such sound.

The development of two qualities of the mind, accelerated by exercise growing out of necessity, has likewise been a boon. These qualities are, first, a visual imagination and, second, a photographic and retentive memory. After twelve sightless years I am still able to see vividly in my mind the physical characteristics and special relationships of any place or room with which I was reasonably familiar during my sighted life. Likewise, with the aid of a graphic, concise and intelligent description (a function in which my wife has been of tremendous assistance), a permanent photographic impression of new rooms or places previously unfamiliar to me is stamped somewhere upon my cerebral cortex to be filed away and used at the proper time. My memory, always sharply photographic and retentive, has proven a major buttress. This quality of memory has served me well in many years, but particularly in the recollection of details concerning patients, in connection with medical literature, and in the memorizing of data for presentation during lectures or clinical papers. There is, of course, a definite and important relationship between the age at which sight is lost and the capacity to develop such physical and mental qualities as I have briefly outlined. The congenitally blind or those becoming so during early childhood have the opportunity to develop their extravisual perceptive functions during the age when aptitude for learning is greatest. I must confess that I sometimes take refuge in such thoughts when I am dispiritedly tempted to compare my own feeble accomplishments with those of persons like Helen Keller, Alec Templeton, Robert Babcock, Woolley, the biological chemist, or Burgess, the naval architect.

Those qualities of the spirit which I like to think may have been stimulated to grow under the influence of my handicap are in some respects so deeply personal that I would hesitate to write about them save under the cloak of anonymity. They are difficult to put into words, but perhaps I may best describe them as an orientation, a putting into proper perspective of the eternal verities, the acquisition of humility and of loving-compassion for mankind, and a riveting in place of my conviction concerning the existence and omnipotence of God. As I sit quietly in the greenish shimmering gloom, the foibles, the foolishness, the greed and cruelty of man recede and assume their proper place. By the faint glow of the tiny inner light which, often waxing and waning, yet never quite goes out, one sometimes fancies that one gains a glimpse of the brooding love and compassion upon the Eternal Face and one knows somehow that we are placed here for a great purpose and that we must struggle to contribute something, however small, to the common good.

Whether or not a by-product of what little increment of the spirit I have achieved, one of my most priceless gifts has been a strengthening of the roots and a burgeoning of the flower of my old friendships. This growth, invisible and yet made tangible in a hundred kind and simple ways, I feel about me as a warm effulgent glow which lights the vista of the years ahead. Nor do such radiations emanate from old friendships alone. There seems an added warmth, a kind of tacit fellowship in my relations now with almost everyone I meet — not the outgrowth of mawkish pity, of superficial sentiment, or of the mere desire to be kind, but an unspoken warmth of feeling which is very real.

Honesty and fairness require an examination of both sides of the coin. What of the rough spots along the road, the stones that bruise the heel and the quag that mires the weary foot? Foremost among those things which most exercise my determination to prevail is a feeling of helplessness or dependence upon others which I suppose besets all those who are blind. Stemming from this is a recurrent self-reproach that I have not kept pace with my mental, emotional and social adjustment. Self-consciousness and embarrassment at public recognition and pity of my handicap have largely faded with the passage of time, but awkward situations often still arise in public places or among crowds which require tact and self-control. Insufficient exercise, and its offspring, insomnia, remain as annoying physical problems. I have become hypersensitive to noise. Though automatically on guard, I still collect my share of tibial, frontal and nasal bruises and cuts. I have been fortunate in escaping major physical injury, but unexpected contact with the edge of an open door remains one of my major hazards.

Despite my best efforts to attain a serenity of spirit, I am still given to outbursts of irritability and to moods of depression during which those I love are most likely to suffer. I own too that I have not been able entirely to overcome my aversion to those people whose efforts at patronizing kindness conceal but poorly the blend of smug pity and repugnance which lies beneath. Greatly to be cherished is the friend who keeps his pity buried deep and whose kindness does not cloy, but is kept faintly acid with the tang of humour and of wit. The indulgence of a sense of humour is of great therapeutic value to those among the sightless so fortunately endowed; Thurber and the *New Yorker* are excellent substitutes for an appointment with a psychiatrist.

So, after twelve years without vision and being now well into my sixth decade, I welcome this opportunity for retrospection, for introspection, and for a summing up of the debits and the credits. It is plain that I have been fortunate, too fortunate perhaps, for the full growth of that toughness of mind and spirit which is essential for the acquisition of maximal independence. Be that as it may, I have much for which to be thankful, blessed as I am with all the benefits of love and friendship, absorbed in congenial work for which I am fitted, possessed of a reasonable degree of economic and academic security; our sons are well on their way through college, and, crowning all these things, there is the consciousness of obstacles overcome. Sometimes I think of that Saul of Tarsus, who, on his way to harry the Nazarenes in Damascus, was blinded by the light of glory so that he might see — and seeing, then became Paul. Thinking of him I know that somewhere there is an answer. For those who may some day stand where I have stood, let these three things be put above price: love, and the privilege of work, and the glow of the little lamp that shines behind the shadow and will never fade.

Chapter IV

# Brown-Séquard Syndrome

This is an account of the development and progress of a neurological syndrome, whose causation has never been firmly
established. It was probably a vascular incident affecting the
cervical spinal cord, probably thrombotic as judged by its slow
onset and progress, but possibly haemorrhagic. One Sunday, I
was pulling horizontally on a rope. Despite the application of
maximum effort for some five minutes, the load could not be
moved until help arrived. The footholds were secure and conveni-
ent, and no bodily distortion was necessary.

No immediate consequences ensued, and later in the day a
steep cliff-path, interspersed with about 100 steps, was mounted
without undue difficulty at a continuous run in competition
with my teenage daughter.

Whether the first (or either) of these incidents was the cause
of the subsequent events is problematical, but they are included
in this account, firstly for completeness, and secondly because I
feel a strong urge to attribute the onset of the illness to a
physical traumatic event, as do most patients.

Not being any longer in the active practice of Medicine, my
job entails office and paper work. Next day, I noticed some
clumsiness and fumbling in the left hand, particularly when trying to manipulate papers. No great thought was given to this at
the time, and other manifestations of impairment of the central
nervous system were neither noted nor sought.

On Tuesday, the dysfunction of my left hand was worse, and
almost caused the enucleation of my eye during the morning
wash (or so it seemed). At work, the fumbling and clumsiness was
obviously worse, and I avoided the use of the left hand whenever
possible. No other symptoms were yet noted, and I was content
at this time to ignore the whole affair.

On Wednesday, I noticed further deterioration during the
morning ablutions. I experienced difficulty in washing the back
of my neck with my left hand. It could be reached, but not with
any degree of accuracy, and that amount of pressure which is
needed to achieve the feeling of being adequately washed, could

not be exerted. A few minutes later, a new sign manifested itself — there was ataxia of the left leg. Since the day before someone had made the stairs steeper and the treads narrower.

Later in the day, I had occasion to scratch myself between the scapulae, at that spot which is just out of reach both from above and from below. For this purpose I usually employ the blunt end of a pencil. On this occasion, I realised that I could not feel the pencil on the right side of the mid-line. This prompted further discreet investigation, and I found an area of pain-loss comprising the right hand, the whole of the arm, and the upper part of the trunk from the shoulder to the level of the umbilicus.

The sensory loss raised some alarm in my mind for the first time. Whilst the motor disturbance was a nuisance, it could be avoided with a modicum of care, but the sensory loss meant loss of protective reflexes and consequent trauma which would be slow to heal. Pictures of neurological classes flooded back to the forefront of the mind, doubtless magnified on their long journey from whatever nooks and crannies of memory where they had been lurking, waiting for just such an opportunity to pounce on my unsuspecting cerebrum.

On Thursday, two incidents impressed on me the extent and the serious nature of my disability. The first occurred during the course of the morning wash. Having first put my right hand into the water, I immersed the left hand — and drew it out again. The water was extremely hot, yet the right hand had not "informed" me of this. Although I was fully aware that pain and temperature sensations are conveyed by similar pathways, and that if one is affected, then the other almost certainly will be too, this discovery was a complete surprise. Naturally, it had to be confirmed by touching various objects, first with one hand, then the other. I found that the hot tap, the cold tap, the bath, the ceiling, and the floor were not merely not hot (or cold) as they should have been, but had no temperature at all. How little, under normal circumstances, we are conscious of the temperature of objects we touch! It only obtrudes into consciousness when the temperature is extreme (either hot or cold) or when it is unexpected. At least, so I found from my left hand during the time when my right hand was hors de combat. It is probably because temperature is so little appreciated that its loss is not realised until an incident like this occurs. When the realisation of the serious consequences which were liable to follow from this sensory loss finally broke down the psychological barrier ("It can't happen to me"), I realised what a precarious position I was in. If the sensory loss had, after all, happened to me, so too could the indolent ulcerations, the burns, the general atrophic changes in the skin, and all the other dire results of sensory loss predicted by my erstwhile neurological tutors who had expounded ad nauseam on this theme with a fervour which would have done credit to an old-time bible-thumping, fire-and-brimstone, revivalist preacher.

When I arrived at work, the car park was empty of people, and it seemed a good opportunity to do a further test. Could I run? Here was smooth level ground, so I broke into a trot. After 3 or 4 paces I had to stop, or fall flat. I stopped. I had been stamping my left foot, the foot did not point in the proper direction but rotated wildly and uncontrollably in all directions, and the leg could not be made to swing in rhythm with its partner.

At this point I had to review my differential diagnosis. Up to now it had consisted of three items: hysteria (heavily favoured), some unknown but self-limiting neurological disorder, and a secondary neoplastic tumour of the cord (site of primary — bronchus). I eliminated the first as being wishful thinking and naive. The second was no longer tenable, as matters were getting worse, and this too, was really only self-deception. This left the third. Well, if it had to be, it had to be. Was it worth doing anything about it? If the disease had progressed to the stage of spinal secondaries, nothing useful could be done anyway, so I may as well die from natural causes, rather than at the hands of my colleagues.

On Friday, nothing new was discovered. The ataxia was worse, and made the negotiation of stairs really difficult, especially going down, but also going up. Because nothing new had happened, I almost reverted to my original diagnosis of hysteria — I had found myself out. It so happens that the external medical adviser for the firm by which I am employed is also my G.P., and he happened to call in today. I mentioned my troubles to him, and after a few quick confirmatory prods and taps, he made arrangements for me to see the local consultant the following morning. I was considerably taken aback at what seemed to me to be undue haste. After all, this was either a hysterical state, a self-limiting condition, or a fatal condition, and therefore could only be of academic interest to anyone.

On Saturday, the consultant not only confirmed my own findings, and delineated them more accurately, but added some new features. Thus, motor function on the right side was also slightly affected, proprioception was missing on the left and deficient on the right, tactile sensations were affected (the milled edge of a half-crown had been smoothed off) on both sides. These new findings startled me — I had not noticed their loss at all. The only regions of my body which were not affected in some way seemed to be the head and neck, yet how little this extensive loss had been noticed.

Arrangements were made for my transfer that day to a neuro-surgical unit some 20 miles away. It was emphasised that this was probably not the most appropriate place to be sent, but in view of the urgency, it would have to do. I could see no reason for urgency, but had a suspicion that other deficiencies had been found which I did not know about. The biggest blow of all fell when I was not allowed to drive myself the 2-3 miles home — I had had no difficulties at all during the week in driving the car. But all protests were brushed aside.

I was transported to hospital by ambulance during the after-noon, exerting my independence and demonstrating my residual capacity by carrying my own meagre luggage myself. I soon found that ward sisters had lost none of their powers of persua-sion since my own hospital days, however, and I was relieved of all loads immediately on entering the ward. I was shown to my bed, and the ward sitting-room was pointed out. Examinations by the house-staff followed and I filled the rest of the day talking to other patients in the sitting-room.

On Sunday, the registrar visited me and was annoyed that I had defied instructions by getting out of bed. Since I had not been given such instructions, I felt rather indignant, not only because of what he said, but also how he said it. I deemed it wise not to argue, but accepted the new instructions to lie still in bed, even to be fed. The feeling of helplessness, hopelessness, frustra-tion and general uselessness which these instructions engendered are quite unimaginable to anyone who has not been subjected to such a régime. Nor were these feelings relieved by the explanation given for their necessity — the risk of total and permanent quadriplegia. A visit from the family later in the day merely emphasised what a vegetable I had become, and how much of a liability I should be to them. Never before or since have I experienced such unremitting gloom and pessimism.

On Monday, the wall by the right side of the bed still had no temperature, and movements of the left arm appeared to be clumsier than ever. An attempt to touch my nose with closed eyes almost caused my transfer to an ophthalmic unit. It was a boring and uneventful day, relieved only by the information that tomorrow I should have a myelogram.

On Tuesday, the wall and the bed-frame were still devoid of temperature, but the tip of my nose has been moved part of the way back to its proper place.

The two porters (Burke and Hare) arrived during the morning to wheel me to the X-ray department for the dreaded myelogram. To anyone else who has to undergo this procedure for the first time, I would say, "Take heart, it really *is* painless. It is not even uncomfortable". Having been replaced on the trolley, and whilst awaiting the arrival of Burke and Hare to take me back to the ward, I was told I was to return the next day to have the contrast medium removed. Despite the ease with which the material had been put in, I did not feel any great enthusiasm about this proposal. After all, I might just have been lucky.

On Wednesday, the wall and the bed-frame were cold! My nose had continued its journey to its proper place and was almost there! But how could this be? The CNS has no capacity for recovery. Having only recently relived all my instruction in neurology, I remembered this fact very well. Was this, after all, merely hysteria? Was this another manifestation of the healing power of the diagnostic X-ray?

Burke and Hare arrived to take me to the X-ray department. Yesterday's lumbar puncture was no fluke — the procedure today was equally devoid of discomfort. During the afternoon, the registrar came to tell me that no abnormality had been discovered on the X-ray, and that I might therefore gradually and gently resume my normal activities. This gave a final boost to my morale which was already high — after all, some recovery was already taking place, and I had twice survived the dreaded lumbar puncture.

On Thursday, I could get up, and I was to go home. The wall and bed-frame were still cold. The washing water had a temperature today too, though it was vague, and was slow to impinge on consciousness. A physiotherapist made me a felt collar which I was to wear for the next month. Later in the day I was driven home, this time by car.

But now a new symptom appeared. On the way home I was gripped by the most ferocious headache. So bad was it that the car had to be stopped so that I could lie down. After about 10 minutes it passed off. This headache was to recur over the next 10-14 days when I at last associated it with the collar. The collar discarded, it did not recur.

Recovery was steady and, apart from the headaches, uneventful. Two weeks after discharge from hospital, I returned to work.

Now, almost three years after this incident, I find I am able to do anything, and feel everything, though not quite normally. For instance, running is still clumsy, my left hand is still a little fumbling, and appreciation of temperature is delayed, so care is needed. For normal activity, both at work, and at play, there is to all intents and purposes, no residual disability.

Several features of this incident have struck me as being worthy of comment since they were so unexpected, and they would cause me to change my approach to patients with neurological disorders. In general, the greatest surprise was in finding how extensive both the motor and the sensory disabilities were before I (as the patient) became aware of them. This applies particularly to the loss of proprioception and the loss of tactile sensation. Possibly work of a more manual nature would have drawn my attention to these disabilities sooner. The second feature is that, although I was fully aware of the possibility of doing myself damage without realising, it still happened. During the period of enforced bed rest, I allowed my finger to stay in a match flame. I was unaware of this until I saw my blackened finger. Fortunately, it was only a deposit of soot, but it might have been worse. I feel now that every neurological lesion merits the demonstration to the patient himself of the dangers which may result from it. Make him run, so that he almost falls; push a large bore needle through a skin-fold and let him watch it being done; hold his finger in a small flame. I think these demonstrations should frighten (not injure) the patient, for only then will he realise the extent of his loss, and the gravity of the situation in which he now finds himself.

I would appeal to physicians to remember, when ordering complete bed rest, that this is a very depressing state to be in. Such orders should not be issued lightly, and only after a full explanation, particularly with respect to the expected duration and the ultimate prognosis, to the patient. As much optimism as is possible, consistent with truth, should be included in this explanation.

Finally, I would ask my colleagues working in hospital to ensure that their orders have been passed on to the patient before admonishing him for not having adhered to instructions. He may well never have received them. Having myself been in this situation, I can assure you that it causes a very great deal of resentment, which may or may not be expressed verbally depending on the personalities of those involved.

Chapter V

# Cancer of the Breast

Symptoms were conspicuous by their absence. I remember thinking to myself, a few months before I discovered the mass, how much older I suddenly felt; that I could not do now what I had done only a year or two before. But then my programme had been a relatively heavy one. The thought that I might be ill certainly never entered my head.

One evening, as I was undressing, I remarked to my husband, a layman — "Gosh I'm getting thin; I can even feel my ribs!". I had touched what I was sure was a rib on my left chest. A month later, while lying in bed, I was horrified to find a large mass there. I have always been rather flat chested, so that missing a lump seems even more surprising. (I never did any self-palpation; I don't think I was ever taught to). Within days, I was in hospital, and had a biopsy and immediate mastectomy. The surgeon remarked to my husband that he didn't know how I could have left it so late — a remark that upset me tremendously. A few months previously, I had seen a gynaecologist for a routine examination and cervical smear. He did not examine my breasts. I was taking an oral contraceptive.

In spite of the seriousness of my illness, a part of my mind was interested in the way I reacted as a patient. At various times since the operation, I have been depressed and agitated, and could not sleep. Partly to pass the time at night, and partly for catharsis, I wrote the following, some eight months after surgery:—

In "The Courage to Be" Tillich describes the three ontological anxieties of man. All three of these I experienced vividly at the time of my operation. First there was blind panic, and the overwhelming feeling that "this can't be happening to me" — this started, of course, before my admission to hospital. In fact, the few days of waiting to go into hospital were in some ways perhaps the worst. This phase is equally present in patients whose lumps in the breast are found, at operation, to be benign! Surgeons should reckon with this anxiety, and neutralise it wherever possible — if necessary, with sedation. When my fears had been confirmed by the biopsy (and immediate mastectomy), there was a lessening of anxiety but a corresponding deepening of despair. Even a few weeks later it seemed strange to me that, having called for a psychiatrist (a former teacher and friend), I greeted her with the statement: "I only want to know how long I have to live!". When she gave some figures — fictitious ones — involving the words "5 years", I looked up in amazement and replied: "But 5 years is a *long* time". I had been reckoning my future in months. This phase corresponds to Tillich's "fear of non-being".

The second phase came later, while I was attending for radio-therapy as an out-patient. I became convinced (for the first time in my life) that God was punishing me, and that I knew why. This phase corresponds to Tillich's "fear of guilt and ultimate condemnation".

The third phase was the most surprising of all. It came still later, and lasted for some months. I was already back at work. Gradually there came upon me a great longing for God, just like the longing for a loved but absent person. I had always loved the first verse of the 42nd Psalm    "As the hart panteth after the water brooks, so panteth my soul after Thee, O God", but I had admired it only for its beauty of language. This was the first time I experienced the feeling it expresses. I was quite familiar with the "Oh, my soul, why art thou cast down?" feeling, but this is a different thing altogether. The longing for God corres-ponds to Tillich's "fear of meaninglessness".

It is generally accepted that anger plays a large part in depres-sion. My case was no exception. Most of my anger was aimed at God, whom I cursed for treating me unfairly. I saw God as a "big bully", and thought: "Why don't You pick on someone of your own strength to fight?". Even animals do not attack weaker individuals of the same species; there is a fish nicknamed "Jack Dempsey", because it is so fair in its fighting. I was reading "On Aggression" by Lorenz at the time, and this accounts for my making comparisons with animals. Lorenz describes the placating gestures in animals, e.g., the rolling over on to its back by a puppy, so that its most vulnerable part, its abdomen, is upper-most, for all the world to see that it has no aggressive intent. In many species of animals, the males and females are distinctly coloured, and a male never attacks a female. However, there is a certain kind of lizard — bright green and pink in colouring — in which the sexes look identical and, in order to protect herself, the female, upon meeting another lizard, makes placating gestures which consist of raising her forelimbs alternately, in a movement reminiscent of piano playing. I thought of myself as such a lizard, despicable and helpless in my placating gestures towards God. I did not tell my psychiatrist of this concept — I discovered that, even with very good rapport, one does not tell one's therapist "everything". The reason for being punished by God I told her only too readily.

Later, of course, I felt guilty at the anger I had felt against God. This was considerably lightened by a passage I read in Lake's "Clinical Theology", to the effect that one may be angry with God, wrestle with Him, even curse Him, as long as one does not forget Him. I now felt that I was possibly underestimating God — surely He is at least as tolerant as the average human parent, who does not reject a child because the child expresses anger on occasion.

I think it is important that someone with sufficient psychological insight and ability to handle the patient's depression and anger, should be available in times of such crisis. I know some of my readers will argue that not every patient becomes as depressed as I was, but I wonder how correct this argument is. Every psychiatric worker knows that, the more frightened a patient is, the less he talks about his fears. Lake points out the need for "an attentive listener who can hear what we cannot put into words, and see what we dare not see ourselves, when the symptoms of the frightened spirit begin to show through in physiognomy or symptom". As Kornfeld wrote "The patient, terrified at having been close to death, may avoid asking questions. Often, the true answers to these unasked questions can be reassuring".

Some readers will be surprised at my preoccupation with religious matters. I had a Calvinistic upbringing, but I am normally not religious. I have long been aware that the mind and body cannot be treated separately. What this illness taught me is that the "mind" and "soul" are equally indivisible.

If depression is not handled adequately, it lasts much longer; and anger is likely to become partly displaced on to other people, including one's medical attendants. I resented the fact that one of my doctors avoided me when I was tearful, but sought me out when I was smiling again. This poor man has to deal exclusively with patients suffering from incurable diseases, and I do not suggest that he can possibly bear all their burdens. What I do think is that someone else (psychiatrically trained) should be included in the team, in order to help.

In discussing attempted suicide, Stengel states that "it sometimes creates the peculiar situation in which somebody who has died and has revived is with us alive while we are mourning him".

The patient with an incurable disease is in a somewhat similar position. He realises that the bell tolls for him — or her — and mourns. There is so much to mourn. I do not feel like Leipoldt, who wrote: "Wat is daar meer deur die dood te rowe? Somer en son en saffier vir my". ("What is there more to be robbed of by death? Summer and sun and sapphire for me"). I have many things and people to mourn. Myself, my husband and children, friends, colleagues, relatives, pets, my home, my work.

I know that depression often follows on the anniversary of a bereavement. What I was not prepared for was a deepening of depression after a visit to a much loved place — in my case, a mental hospital where I had worked, and where I have many friends on the staff.

Women who have not had children, or who have not yet married, can be expected to be deeply depressed after mastectomy, as their losses become more immediate and more final.

If oophorectomy is carried out as well as mastectomy, the patient has, of course, a precipitate menopause to deal with too — one that may not be completely alleviated with hormones.

Since undergoing mastectomy, I have been preoccupied with poetry and music concerned with mourning — especially Hiawatha's beautiful lament, and one stanza from the Rubaiyat of Omar Khayyam (Fitzgerald):—

> "Lo! Some we loved, the loveliest and the best
> That Time and Fate of all their Vintage prest,
> Have drunk their Cup a round or two before,
> And one by one crept silently to Rest".

Like Captain Cat in Dylan Thomas' "Under Milkwood", I have thought of my dead friends, especially of two women who were both younger than I at the time of their death; both had young children. At such times I am grateful that I still have the good fortune to be alive.

The mastectomy patient has to mourn the loss of her physical completeness — the loss of a breast and of a normal unswollen arm. She realises at last that she is no longer young. As she takes leave of her low-cut dresses, she also takes leave finally of youth with its shining hopes, and of the phantom figures of her first loves. She needs help with a prosthesis. I floundered without this at first and ran the gamut of embarrassing experiences because of the absent breast — looking deformed, feeling uncomfortable, and being quite unable to get clothes to fit properly. It is not necessary for women in this day and age to have to wear in their "bra" such things as cotton wool, bird seed, beads, or plastic chips in little bags. Excellent prostheses are available. It is, however, essential that the prosthesis be brought to the patient, whose depression makes it impossible for her to go and look for one.

Looking back at the post-operative period, I feel that my doctors should have talked to me about my illness. My surgeon was silent and glum. The G.P. in the picture was busy and a stranger to me. The radiotherapist, from whom I expected most support, was quite incapable of talking to me when I most needed it. He studiously avoided me when I was depressed, and I resented this. Is there such a thing as "third-week blues?". The radiographers glibly talked of it. If it were not for the psychiatrist, I do not know how I would have got through that period. I also remember with gratitude the attitude of the nursing sister in the psychiatric ward, where I had once worked, when I went to her weeping, saying: "I've come for some first-aid". One of the radiographers endeared herself to me when she assured me it was "still early days". In contrast, another radiographer seemed even more anxious and upset than I was — this did not help me at all! I resented the radiotherapist's adjective "fabulous" to describe my mastectomy scar.

I did not suffer from pity for myself only. After my 5 weeks of deep therapy, I went back to hospital for another biopsy and oophorectomy. During this stay I was much concerned with the emotional welfare of a fellow-patient, a recent immigrant, who was in a state of near panic as she waited all morning to go to the theatre without any sedation. I could not help but compare this patient's handling with the superb way in which an ophthalmologist treated an apprehensive old lady who was to have a cataract removed. He sedated her so heavily pre-operatively that I was afraid she might get hypostatic pneumonia. However, the ophthalmologist was obviously right, for many hours after the operation (which was done under local anaesthesia), the patient woke up and asked when she would be going for surgery. Nor did she get pneumonia!

I have moved to a different part of the country, and so have a new radio-therapist. Fortunately, my new doctor knows how to deal with me as a whole person, and not merely as an illness. I feel confident that he will be able to support me through whatever difficult times may lie ahead. I cannot express my gratitude to him adequately. Suffice it to say that, although my disease has progressed, I can face the future with an equanimity quite unknown to me previously. This man has mastered the very difficult art of inspiring calm and confidence, even while not being quite dishonest about a potentially sinister disease. In the final analysis, I think it is a doctor's personality structure and motivation (and not his training) which determine whether he will be merely a good technician or a doctor in the fullest sense of the word.

What a heavy burden doctors took upon themselves when they took over the care of the sick from the priests and diviners. One could insert into the Hippocratic Oath something like the following:— "I undertake to play the role of God for my patient when the latter so desires me to do", for a patient with a serious illness regresses to an infantile state of mind and expects his doctor to play the role of mother — and an infant's mother is its whole universe, including its God. Masserman has written of "the Ur delusions" one of which is "the delusion of the omnipotent servant" whereby we paradoxically expect God, who is omnipotent, to do our bidding in all things. If this is an impossible demand, how much more impossible is often a patient's expectation of his doctor, who is not even omnipotent.

Another of the "Ur delusions" is that of man's immortality. No-one can really accept that he will cease to exist. When this delusion is severely shaken so also is the patient. A psychologist with long experience often protests: "I am not the bluebird of happiness", yet that is, of course, exactly the expectation his patients have of him. My present doctor has warned me that "the honeymoon" will not last. He says his patients shower him alternately with gratitude and insult. I can understand that. I myself would like very much never to see the man again; my dependence on him is too painful a reminder of my plight. It is as if death stands behind him, and some of the horror one feels for that grim spectre must at times rub off on to the doctor, who is seen as the only one between us. Read again Axel Munthe's description of his enemy, death; every good doctor surely echoes his sentiments. Even in more everyday situations it is apparent that people do not enjoy feeling indebted to each other. My husband expresses this truth well; he says:— "If you do anyone a favour, he will never forgive you".

I was 38 when I had my mastectomy in Sept. 1968. In July, 1969, I developed a gland in the neck on the side opposite the tumour. In April 1970 I developed skin secondaries. At this time, I became very depressed and was thinking of suicide, though only for a later date. I consulted a G.P. about my death. It was the first time I had consulted him; I had not needed a G.P. before. He asked me about my faith; I said I had none. Without telling me, he asked for special prayers for me at a nearby monastery. Just over a week later I met again for the first time in 24 years a childhood friend, Dr. B., who is a minister of religion and a recently qualified doctor. We talked a lot about life, death and immortality. I had never been able to conceive of eternity, and did not believe in life after death. For me, life has sometimes only been bearable because of the thought that one could always remove yourself from it if things got too bad. Dr. B., on the other hand, only found this life worth living because there was something else beyond it. I said I would die willingly if only there was "a meaning". Dr. B. talked against suicide and atheism. I had planned to have no funeral service whatever; he said he would be willing to hold one for me. Suddenly my mood turned to elation. I am 40 years old and have never been elated before, though often depressed.

I live at a coastal resort to which Dr. B. had come for a short holiday. After he left, my mood rose even higher, and I could not sleep at all. At the same time, I began to suffer from a formal thought disorder such as one finds in early schizophrenia. Everything had a symbolic meaning, and had a message for me. It was all very funny. My husband took me to a psychiatrist, who ordered a tranquilliser. However, I insisted on admission to an open psychiatric ward, where I stayed for 5 days. After this, I was well enough to go back to work. The thought disorder and elation had both subsided.

Dr. B. had said he would be coming back in September, and had promised that we would "paint the town red". All was well with me emotionally for the next few months, but in September I became restless and excitable again, and could not sleep. Dr. B. did not come. The thought disorder returned, and I requested readmission. This time the thought disorder seemed less pleasant to me, and I wanted it to stop. I felt like the Sorcerer's apprentice. I again recovered within days on a tranquilliser, and after a fortnight was mentally well and back at work.

I find the following passage from Herzberg's "Work and the Nature of Man" very significant: "The need to synthesize psychological input is as important to man as is the need of the centipede to unify the action of all of his legs in order to walk. Man will disintegrate psychologically if he is unable to cope with the tremendous amount of information that he receives and if there is no possibility of giving the data some unified meaning."

## Chapter VI

# Cardiac Valve Replacement

Nine and a half weeks ago my mitral valve was replaced with an aortic homograft transplant and on my return to work last week a surgical colleague begged me to commit to writing my memory of the ordeal before it became faded or distorted. He said, furthermore, that surgeons were eager to know and understand more about the reactions of patients who had undergone surgery of this severity. I should point out that cardiothoracic surgery is not my line of country and that I am only a gynaecologist. My knowledge, such as it is, of modern cardiology has been acquired only recently in the course of intensive study while in hospital and from personal experience.

Eight years ago I had undergone mitral valvotomy, an experience which horrified me far more than I had expected, and it was therefore with some apprehension that I faced a second thoracotomy, but the sheer misery of acute congestive cardiac failure drove me to change my mind, if only as an act of suicide. A large and very tender liver made getting in and out of a car hateful and pulmonary congestion and hypertension had wrecked most nights' sleep over nearly two years. I repeatedly found myself reciting Keats' lines: "Now more than ever seems it rich to die . . ."

### Cardiac Catheterisation and
### Angiocardiography

I found this worse than I had expected. The department itself was impressive in the electronic sense with television-viewing screens wherever I looked unless I kept my eyes shut. Spreadeagled on the angiocardiographic table for what seemed a very long time I was well aware that at any moment ventricular fibrillation might be my lot and took somewhat cold comfort from the knowledge that D.C. defibrillators were instantly available and that my colleagues, now buzzing around me, would hardly be disturbed if they had to put the drill into effect. I made a little speech about being basically neurotic and on overhearing the level of my pulmonary-artery pressure and commenting thereat I quickly realised I had better keep silent and not upset everyone.

The passage of the catheters both femoral and brachial was not in itself painful, merely peculiar, and the injection of various radio-opaque dyes momentarily put the brain on fire, then the pelvis and curiously the glans penis and finally the hands and feet, as though the sheer heat ran out of one. I was aware of great satisfaction amongst my colleagues investigating me and the fact that some of the tests were repeated more than once I attributed to their enthusiasm over their success, rather than to a bad result in the first place. At the end of it all the elbow of my friend, the senior radiologist, was applied with bar-counter precision to my femoral pressure point while a number of pleasantries were exchanged. On return to the ward the trouble really started, with acute pelvic pain and retention of urine, doubtless aggravated by the diuretic effect of some of the radio-opaque dyes. The procedure had been undertaken under the full influence of warfarin, so I was alert for signs of residual bleeding and presently felt a double mass in my own pelvis through the abdominal wall. I suspect that my enthusiastic colleagues were not at first convinced that I was developing a retroperitoneal haematoma tracking up into the pelvis, and I had the subsequent satisfaction of proving that I was right by going over to a neighbouring hospital with the necessary equipment and getting an ultra-sonogram taken, which demonstrated it well. I immediately had copies made together with slides for my next American lecture on the subject of ultrasonics and was able to pull the legs suitably of my radiological friends.

An anxious and depressing 36 hours ensued while the computer spewed back the results. My beloved physician-in-chief, almost with tears in his eyes, opined that it would be monstrous not to give me a new of reconditioned mitral valve. Both he and the surgeon of my choice (and incidentally his) soon convinced me of the benefit of a human cadaver aortic valve in place of my own worthless mitral, mainly because of the reduced risk of embolism, of which I was in some dread, and because a burst of tachycardia, provoked by the many silly things that happen in my sort of life, would not precipitate the acute kind of failure encountered with plastic prostheses.

I now began involuntarily but doggedly to acquire all the information I could about the operation I was about to undergo, even pumping information out of nurses who had worked in the cardiac theatres, although I must say that both surgeons and physicians did all they could to forewarn me and therefore to forearm me with what to expect.

## Was it a good thing to be a doctor?

I have not the slightest doubt about this. Sufficient familiarity
and understanding of the theme even made grim jesting possible.
I encountered one or two patients, lay people in the ward, who
took an entirely different view, did not wish to know which
valve was being replaced or why, and more or less begged to be
spared any details of their forthcoming operation. I am now convinced, however, that the more a patient knows about the details,
why and wherefore of his operation, the better; above all, what
to expect in the way of postoperative symptoms. I was warned,
for example, not to undertake too elaborate an examination of
my own central nervous system after a prolonged period on
cardiopulmonary bypass. This certainly prevented panic in the
first few postoperative days, when I found my intention tremor
almost uncontrollable and which might otherwise have led to a
rapid surmise that there had been some neurological damage.

## The operation itself

Two very merry anaesthetists visited me on several occasions and
helped me with a little whisky which I had tucked away in my
locker. Soon our attitude showed signs of hilarity. The number
of preoperative samples of blood, X-rays, bacterial swabs, urine
specimens, and so on, soon outpaced the list of tests to which I
thought laboratories could be put, but then, as stated before, I
am only a simple gynaecologist. By now I was reasonably out of
cardiac failure and able to take a much more focused view of life
and to some extent of death as well.

The premedication was obviously a success and I was merely
aware of going in and out of lifts, of gates closing and opening,
behind and in front of me, and of the ceiling lights in the anaesthetic room. I had just enough time to admonish the anaesthetists
suitably and frivolously of the dangers of intra-arterial injections
when they mastered my insolence with their drugs and the next
five hours' work was begun.

## Intensive-care unit

I woke up, it was still daylight, and, as expected, I found a tube
in my trachea. I greeted my wife momentarily, observed her dress,
and it is said I embraced the sister of the department on both
cheeks, but of this I have no recollection, so can give no opinion
as to whether this was instinct, habit, or mistake. There seemed
to be an awful lot of tubes going in and out of me in all sorts of

sites and directions, including a catheter in my bladder, for which I felt grateful as I had feared postoperative retention, and in spite of a good deal of practice with a urine bottle in bed preoperatively felt far from confident that I would be able to micturate spontaneously. This had bothered me rather a lot and I had warned the doctors beforehand.

I started moving fingers and toes as a start to an examination of my own neurological system, but did not get very far before the next injection of Omnopon turned my life into a blank once more. Pain was not the main feature of my remembered experiences at this stage. From now on brief glimpses of consciousness were quickly suppressed, again I believe with Omnopon, even before I had time to clamour for it or express gratitude or the reverse.

I now began to feel a great sense of frustration and annoyance at being unable to communicate because of the presence of the endotracheal tube. I signalled for writing materials but nobody understood. I was evidently now past the curare stage but if I have any recollection at all of being ventilated under the influence of curare and under no control of my own, I can only say that it did not terrify me as I had expected it to; in fact, on one occasion the respirator tube came adrift and I felt two blasts of air in my face and had just long enough to think, with dismay more than panic, that I had succeeded in disconnecting myself before I was immediately reconnected. I was grateful, in fact, that the respirator was doing my breathing for me and was soon asleep again.

My awareness of dehydration was intense and one of the most unpleasant features that I can recall at this time was the dry, rasping bandage stuffed between my teeth and across the roof of my mouth whose function was clearly to hold the endotracheal tube in place. For a wild and wicked moment I considered chewing my way through it with my teeth but had enough sense not to carry out the plan. Even after an anaesthetic the mouth would appear to be a very sensitive area.

A rather thrusting young nephew of mine, now working at another hospital as a medical registrar, came to see me, donned a gown and barged in, in front of everybody. I can remember, as can others, my vituperative comments in vivid but hardly printable language. He obeyed my instructions and rapidly disappeared.

Of the three days spent in the intensive-care unit the third was easily the worst. By now I was conscious for a good deal of the time and much more aware of pain. My endotracheal tube was out and all my drains had been removed. I had greatly feared the pain of removing drains, especially from the pleural cavities, recalling very vividly the removal of such a drain after my valvotomy years ago; in fact I can still hear in my imagination the undignified yell which I uttered on that occasion. It is said that I reacted very unhappily to the procedure this time but I have no recollection of it whatsoever, for which I am very thankful. The sound of one's own voice yelling in acute pain is a demeaning and unnerving experience. The torture chambers of history and indeed of the present must be full of such harrowing incidents.

I remember removing my own catheter, although whether this was official or not I cannot say. My back ached and my buttocks were very sore and, in fact, developed pressure sores at this time. I mentioned the Scottish trick of using a sheepskin rug when nursing patients with vulnerable pressure points and my surgeon promptly disappeared for about twenty minutes and came back with one. He said he had been to Australia and shot it.

I overheard remarks that I was to be transferred back to my ward and my impatience became very great.

### Return to the ward

This was almost like a return in triumph. The welcome of the sister and the nursing staff was certainly heartwarming. There was a good deal of badinage about not being got rid of so easily as all that. My pleasure, however, began to fade as the pain in my chest increased. This was something I had not been warned about in advance. A midsternal split is clearly a very painful incision and it begins to feel really bad about nine or ten days after the operation and now began to discharge fluid copiously from a number of sites. It seemed to me, at least, that my bones were not knitting and I began to fear luridly that I would get a "burst chest" rather like some of my patients in the past have developed burst abdomens. After a day of envisaging what I would look like with my sternum fallen apart I was finally reassured by the surgeons that they had never seen this happen yet. The pain of breathing was considerable and that of coughing indescribable. The prevention of a sneeze had all the features of an ugly emergency.

### Physiotherapists

In retrospect I feel very sorry for these dedicated women who are so determined that one will not end up crippled with flexion deformities of the spine and unable to use shoulders or arms or even straighten the neck, quite apart from the difficulties of

pulmonary expansion of which, fortunately, I had none, thanks
to giving up the dirty habit of smoking ten years ago. I have seen
men groan, mentally at least if not out-spokenly, at the physio-
therapists' entry into the ward and somehow I was glad of any
excuse not to be put through my paces. It was only presently
when I began to realise my appalling limitation of shoulder and
neck movements that I began to take their exercises and antics
more seriously. The term "physioterrorist" is understandable in
the first few postoperative days, but hardly excusable. I unkindly
asked my own physiotherapist if she had even had one of her
patients break to pieces in her hands, or if an arm which she had
been manipulating had ever come away from the patient, and
she took the taunts in remarkably good part. To see me now
driving a car·and sailing a small dinghy, less than ten weeks after
my operation, would give her cause for pride in her handiwork.

## Nursing Care

Being of a susceptible nature I soon found myself adoring all my
nurses, both individually and collectively. For instance I soon
got myself out of bed to tease them rather than because of my
own belief in early ambulation. It was almost a point of honour
not to trouble them for a bedpan, or to ring the bell for anything
that was not distressingly urgent, like the filthy mess I was con-
tinually getting into with the copious discharge from various
sites in my wound. This discharge was a curious dark, mahogany-
coloured fluid, non-purulent and at one stage it got so bad that
the ward sister applied a colostomy bag and amounts of up to
150 ml. at a time were pumped out of it with a syringe. Disaster,
however, overtook me on the second night when the bag burst
in my bed and everything had to be changed. I accused my
precious surgeon jocularly with having done the wrong operation
by mistake and of having performed a colostomy, but he, with
aplomb equal to the occasion, gave it as his opinion that the fluid
looked much more biliary than faecal. I began to realise at this
stage that nobody was likely to take me very seriously and everyone seemed irritatingly confident in my recovery.

About this time I began to receive a number of "slap you on
the back" type of letters from colleagues who wrote that they
expected any minute now to be run off their feet by my new-
found activity, whereas those who counselled me to take life
easily from now on irritated me even more. It was obviously time
for me to be on my way and three and a half weeks after my
operation I took my leave and started on a course of convales-

cence which proved so strenuous, including the launching and commissioning of a small cruiser yacht on the South Coast of England that I decided to return to my own department for a rest.

## Conclusion

For a patient undergoing this type of surgical ordeal morale is clearly paramount. Psychologically I think I have come out of this operation less scathed than after my first thoracotomy, partly because, although I feared it, I knew what to expect, and the general attitude around me was not one of caution about how I should conduct my future life, but one of almost reckless encouragement to do anything I chose. To one who had been trying to live ever more cautiously within a diminishing cardiac reserve over the past few years, this was a refreshing change of attitude. I was delighted to watch the same attitude at work in the case of other cardiac lesions, not necessarily surgical. Perhaps the days are not so far off when other members of the profession will follow the splendid example of this unit in which I was privileged to be treated, in which patients instead of being told to take things easily are clearly encouraged to live their lives to their fullest capacity.

A patient may indeed be calculatingly grateful for the diagnostic, surgical and nursing skill which he has received but to leave hospital with a new and constructive attitude to yet another period of bonus time counts for even more.

# Chapter VII

# Cervical Spondylosis

In 1943 — I was then 33 — I had repeated an old skiing injury of the left knee (internal cruciate ligament) and had been posted to a rather quiet job. I was anxious to prove that the leg was all right and went round a kind of obstacle course, jumped short off my bad leg, missed my next footing and went head first into a lump of iron. I got my left hand to it first and then made violent contact with my left malar bone. I did not knock myself out, but vomited soon after, and feeling shaken put myself to bed, which I do not usually do. The next morning I was examined and found to have a cracked head of radius and a bruised face. The point of contact was anaesthetic over a small area for some months and then developed protopathic sensation which has since disappeared. I was looked upon as a case of concussion, though I remember only wondering at first whether I had broken my jaw. A neurologist, whom I saw six weeks later when I was posted to the Middle East, thought I had had a mild cerebral contusion.

I had headaches, chiefly frontal, and a feeling of woolliness and unsteadiness, particularly with travelling over rough roads or if I did anything with force, a thing I would normally enjoy. I also had a low pitched tinnitus appearing slightly left of centre, which was also accentuated by effort. Most harmful was bending the head forward for a time, or lifting things high in front of me. The symptoms did not usually start till after a delay, sometimes of seconds but usually of some minutes (?spasm ?swelling) and then went through one or more phases of development. But I would emphasise that the "prodromal" phase (if one could call it so, as it could last weeks) was the worst, the period of undefined instability and vagueness, associated with a feeling of slight pressure or void at the back of the throat, possibly extending down towards the thorax. Language here is inevitably vague as one is describing a sensation which seems barely connected with the ordinary senses. There may or may not be also mild aching in the back of the neck, but whatever the cause there was an accompanying vagueness, much as one might have from physical shock. The development of the moderate headache was in fact an improvement.

Later my wife could spot these from the sagging of the facial muscles. I made attempts to break out by persuading myself that this was hysteria or depression at first, and using my full strength, but that only increased the backlog of symptoms to be worked through. I did about eighteen months travelling up Italy. The Anzio Beachhead where I arrived after the first major fighting had died down was far preferable to my last job with 5th Corps because there was much less distance to travel, in jeeps instead of hard sprung trucks, and I had a considerable build up of headaches in the last job. I eventually went sick and was sent to see a neurologist in Naples, who perhaps out of kindness advised repatriation to the Oxford Head Injury Hospital. I think it fair to say that I was not regarded as a crock, because I was offered promotion to 8th Army H.Q. if I would stay.

At Oxford no special examination of my neck was made, perhaps in view of my original notes classing me as a head injury, and in any case their load of severe cases was very considerable. I had by this time learnt to avoid symptoms, and there were none obvious to see. I played tennis indifferently as running produced symptoms, and I gave up P.T. after unpleasant sequelae, but I could always do things at a cost. An eminent neuropsychiatrist suggested that I was suffering from depression. When I went to him eighteen months later saying things were no better, he said I was not now depressed, but had developed anxiety hysteria. I did not take his advice to see a psychiatrist. I also showed him an X-ray of my neck taken at Charing Cross Hospital, which was said to show an abnormal third cervical vertebra, but he judged this irrelevant. Re-entering civilian life my great difficulty was with bending the head for reading and writing and bending over patients to examine them. I adopted various positions such as chin propping, as far as possible. All forms of hard exercise, which I had previously enjoyed, were impossible except gentle skiing and half power swimming without diving. One day I had been carrying our child on my head and found later that my legs were weak, working the car pedals. I went to a rheumatologist who regarded the condition as cervical spondylosis.

Over the last twenty-seven years there have been continuous ups and downs. There is always a tendency after a good spell to hope the thing has stopped and make one of the "dangerous" movements, which could then precipitate the whole process. More recently I have awakened in the morning with symptoms that would get better as the day went on. (Differential diagnosis, Depression!).

A symptom which seemed to produce medical incredulity was

sensitiveness to engine vibration. Soon after being demobilised I found that a six-cylinder car built up a continuous headache, whereas a four might not. A new engine tends to be worse for a while as it gets looser and then enters its good phase, which might then disappear suddenly, say 12,000 miles onward. This has meant considerable expense and experience in trying out all sorts of cars. My present one, though not absolutely the best, has remained tolerable for much longer — till quite recently. Then the choke cable broke and I did not realise that for some time the engine was running on a very weak mixture, producing a different beat. It seems this is not a question of absolute smoothness versus roughness, but of certain periodicities and I cannot necessarily detect them. A car may feel good but build up a headache. Equally, once the cord, if that is what it is, is sensitised it is not easy to know if one is dealing with the original trauma or new stimuli. As for other travel, buses are bad because of hard suspension and often quite vicious stopping. Tubes are acceptable provided I can travel backwards, as this avoids the tendency for the head to flex when stopping.

I have had various pains over the shoulders and higher up the neck in the usual way. They shift, sometimes taking weeks or months, and easily come back to the same position. I have also been treated for a right tennis elbow with intra-articular cortisone. This seemed partly effective, but the pain went when I changed the car, which had heavy steering. Nevertheless, it was quickly succeeded by bilateral tender first carpo-metacarpal joints and this seemed to me suspicious, as these were succeeded by a tender right deltoid muscle on occasion reverting to the wrist again. I had other tender spots on the end of fingers, with nothing abnormal apparently there. But with the carpo-metacarpal joints I could swear there was slight swelling on the right side and a feeling of grating, and it had come after heavy digging. Is there a possibility that a nerve pressure induced tenderness can be associated with trophic change?

A further light on development came at a later stage. When lying in bed (and I once detected a similar state as I came out of a bad dream) I found myself in the severe "prodromal" stage, but as I moved to a different position the right deltoid pain would change to a less well developed left deltoid pain or track down to a pain in the hand. Equally, the "prodromal" stage with its feeling of inner instability might travel forward, as it had done in earlier severe phases, from the back of the throat to a feeling of swelling of the lips and of salivation at the corner of the mouth. On other occasions there seemed a fairly quick development from the lower end of the sensation into what might be the mediastinum, with a feeling of breathlessness and a bounding kind of pulse, not necessarily quicker. This seemed to me to be of too short a duration and too dissociated to be an expression of tension.

A more chronic manifestation which could be connected is that for some years now my swallow mechanism has been less reliable; a little saliva almost automatically being swallowed, enters the glottis. Of course, this mechanism misfires with most people, but at around twice a week this is far above my previous average.

The sensation of slight leg weakness, usually right, reappears from time to time, soon after some traumatic activity, and usually goes off in a few hours to a few days. It appeared regularly for some years after a journey over a rough stretch of road. When it has been more severe, there has been at times a sensation of tremor, about 3-4 a second, of fairly short duration. I doubt whether any tremor was visible. I would say that continuous activity such as gardening (without stooping and pulling up resistant plants) seems to have a good effect, as does persistent vibration, e.g. a car journey that begins with symptoms seems to shake things into place sometimes. Equally, a continuous engine vibration of the traumatic kind has produced new symptoms, or a tenderised state in which new ones are precipitated. The tinnitus has lasted for long periods, but until the most recent episode had become much less. One thing which could indicate its nature, which I have only recently noticed, is that turning the head to the left when lying down has actually stopped it or made it intermittent, and I have been able to repeat this several times on one occasion. Unfortunately on other occasions the effect was less certain, and anyway the position was uncomfortable.

One last symptom has developed, a clicking in the neck with each inspiration in certain positions, when lying down, but perhaps because I change position, I have not noticed any bad effect from it.

Various treatments were tried during exacerbations, but usually after I had waited some weeks in case the symptoms went. I have luckily never had the very severe pain some people have. I have had neck traction up to 400 lbs with manipulation: one cannot fail to be impressed with this and want to report improvement. I have also tried traction by hanging in a collar: this gives a fair sensation of relief till the traction is released. Also, beyond a certain point it seems to reprecipitate instability.

A collar was found not to fit. The chief of my department had already been anxious about it and I also had my doubts about patients seeing it, and it was not worn for long. I had already discussed with the rheumatologist the question of steadying the head at night. Wrapping a towel round the neck did not work, but lying on one's back with neck flat and a pillow each side of the head did work in my case, once I had learnt to sleep on my back (and snore). I also have at times produced greater extension by pulling the mattress five inches beyond the head of the bed, so that the head sank back further. Though there may have been local improvement with other methods, it has seemed to me that the dividend from the last precautionary measure was far the greatest. There was a considerable relief of the muzziness which used to persist for long periods and my tolerance of the "dangerous" activities increased, but this position could be accompanied by mild pain in the left scapula. It must be admitted though that at the same time I had given up one job, roughly halving my town driving. The tinnitus now rarely noticed except after considerable effort.

Perhaps I should add that since puberty I have developed a minor kyphoscoliosis which later showed slight vertebral wedging on X-ray. This has never interfered much with my activity, but could have produced a greater neck lordosis, and possibly other effects. I also developed lumbar symptoms of a mild degree in my late forties. Again I do not think this was anything remarkable, except that I do believe that injection of dextrose solution to produce fibrosis round the vertebra had some steadying effect, and contrary to usual advice a flat bed produces great stiffness before morning. I sleep in a saggy bed across a folded towel in the lumbar region.

Since writing this account I have had to eat my words, which I suppose is typical of the condition. I lifted a fairly heavy hurdle, not perhaps so prophylactically to the side of me as I had hoped, and experienced no serious effect, but presumably something had moved or compressed, as when later I drove the car which had developed the unfavourable vibration, and later did some stooping peering at the mixture control on the carburettor, I had a relapse with the usual "prodromal" symptoms, plus mild weakness in both legs, chiefly quadriceps, and for the first time in the left arm, mainly triceps, but obviously things were fairly loose as there were various shifts. I also developed a sensation of giddiness without rotation lasting two to three hours. I wondered if the precipitation in an already softened field was due not only to the stooping but bending the head back to see the carburettor.

I have only had giddiness twice before, once when doing stiff P.T. at Oxford Head Injury Hospital, and six months ago a rather different experience for no apparent reason while driving, a sensation of severe giddiness lasting only two or three seconds but repeated about fifteen seconds later. Each time I wondered whether I had swerved the car.

The favourite position of lying supine in bed with flat neck no longer worked — in fact it produced further pressure effects. After about three weeks improvement, loss of muzziness and less persistent other symptoms, had begun, and with a kind of sanguine impatience which I should have recognised, I started trying to pull out a stake, in front of me, which is a bad position. There followed a more severe relapse, including inability to find any position in bed where sensations did not accumulate, including the supine one, but I eventually tried the version of this with greater neck extension. This surprisingly slowly produced relaxation. As a therapeutic manoeuvre, however, it obviously only suits some situations out of apparently similar ones, and only in one person and that in the face of mechanically lessened front to back measurement in the spinal canal. I feel the supine position with side support to the head remains prophylactic, if it can be maintained, but one has to distinguish between the effects of (a) avoidance of flexion, (b) avoidance of unchecked movements in sleep, and (c) extra extension, in a condition which may be relatively stationary or gradually advancing.

To sum up, what I call the "prodromal" stage is misnamed. It is clearly the early acute stage of injury whether it causes swelling or vascular spasm, but I suspect the doctor tends to see a later stage or at least the history is coloured by the more concrete manifestations.

The points that strike me are:

a) the difficulty of diagnosis if the symptoms are out of the ordinary: in any case they may shift considerably.

In my own practice I have cases referred where there may be neurotic sensations or mild disc symptoms which have produced reactive tension or depression, and these may be increased by a lack of medical certainty or unawareness of the patient's problem. The examining clinician for his part seems appalled at the overlay or nervous history and is only too glad to get the case off his hands — understandably I would admit in some cases. The more straightforward ones I hold on to, doing little more than giving what explanation I can, with or without a monoamine oxidase inhibitor and tranquilliser, hoping for the likely remission.

b) the importance of the early phase, to me at any rate, with the feeling of deep physical unease (as opposed to psychological) and difficulty of description and the corresponding need for a medical man, who can make sense of the phenomena. Particularly the mental effects, which I do not think are all psychological, the lip sensations, tinnitus and possible mediastinal involvement.

c) the apparent independence of some symptoms, apparently arthritic, which yet succeed each other, possibly repeatedly, and the remarkable phase experienced in bed when the situation appears to be fluid and there is a tentative change-over between symptoms. And

d) the possible importance, anyway prophylactically, of head position at night.

One morning when I started to shave, the soap stick fell from my left hand, I then found I could not hold it between my thumb and fore finger: then I discovered I could not abduct or adduct thumb and fingers, but I could fully flex and extend them; that is, I had full power of grasping and had not any other signs or symptoms of illness and was quite well. In a few days, perhaps a week, I found the same condition was developing in my right hand. Soon all the intrinsic muscles of both hands were paretic — I do not use the word "paralysed" as, to my thinking, paralysis implies permanency — and atrophy was developing, obviously, in the interossei and lumbricales. I had no pain nor any sensory disturbance: nor any diminution of the flexor or extensor power of fingers.

In two years I had complete recovery of all the paretic muscles and of the atrophy.

I was seen by the hospital consultant physician and attended the physiotheraphy department, for these two years, on three days a week, receiving the usual treatment, hot wax, baths, radiant heat, diathermy and interrupted galvanic current applied to each muscle.

All this time I kept at work, was never ill and never had any pain. The only inconvenience was that small change would drop through my fingers and in using knife or fork my forefinger would slip off the instrument.

In about seven or eight months, one day, while applying the current, I suddenly found I could move my right forefinger sideways! That was a great occasion, and this sign of recovery progressed slowly until I had full abduction and adduction in all the small muscles of both hands, and the hollows between the bones filled up again until complete recovery came.

X-rays of my neck showed much arthritic change — cervical

spondylosis. This condition has never caused me any trouble, beyond an occasional stiff and creaking neck.

The text books and many papers I have since read all stress that pain is the first symptom of pressure from bone on the spinal nerves: then will follow sensory signs. Of these I never had any.

The only treatment of any use was the interrupted galvanic current, applied by myself 30 times to each individual muscle at a sitting; the others were really a waste of time and money. The current kept the atrophied muscles alive until the motor nerves transmitted again the stimulus to contract.

Chapter VIII

# Cholecystectomy

Kind gentlemen, your pains
Are register'd where every day I turn
The leaf to read them.
*Macbeth*, 1, 3.

My pain began after a delicious Sunday lunch of roast pork with
all the trimmings — epigastric, continuous, a feeling of most
painful distension, quite unresponsive to any stimulus such as
antacids, a hot drink, or change of posture. Associated flatulence,
with air-swallowing and belching, bringing great expressions of
sympathy from the rest of the family, presumably indicated
associated pylorospasm. There had been two previous attacks in
past months with some fatty dyspepsia in between, bringing the
first small rift in fifteen years of married bliss, because dishes
that had reached the height of culinary perfection were incrimin-
ated. Dark suggestions had been made that it was time for an
X-ray, which I had resisted on the twin assumption that a surgeon
could never really have any of the conditions which he treated
daily, and that my pain was obviously due to a minor cause, such
as gastric allergy, oesophageal regurgitation, or intestinal colic.

But this time things were different. It soon became obvious
that there was to be no easy release. A nonchalant but determined attempt to relive the age of elegance with a large plate of
artichoke soup followed by an evening cigar was crowned by
redoubled agony. Twenty-four hours' further suffering brought
me, tail between my legs, to my radiological colleague, with the
fading hope that it might all turn out to be neurotic. The fervent
hope for a normal cholecystogram obviously illustrated an
intellectual obscurantism partly toxic in origin; for what other
dread cause might then have to be investigated? But a non-
functioning gallbladder clinched the diagnosis.

The problem of management now arose. After much thought
I decided to cancel all professional commitments, only to find
this had already been done by my assistants. The corollary was
to go home rather chastened, and place myself in the hands of
my family doctor, who was, in fact, waiting at home to take
over. A short frank talk resulted in agreement that most attacks

of biliary colic settle in a few hours, and operation could be planned in the next few weeks. This simple plan was vitiated by the intensity of the pain continuing through the third day into the fourth, and reducing 14 stones of prime manhood to abject jelly. By this stage morphine gr. $\frac{1}{3}$ was bringing two hours of partial relief. My family doctor was also feeling the need of relief, and admission to hospital for emergency cholecystectomy was arranged on the fourth day.

The ambulance journey to hospital, with symptoms reaching a crescendo, was only mitigated by the calm and confidence appearance of my senior colleague. The necessary course of action was shown to be quite obvious, and arrangements had already been made. My progress, to the anaesthetic room seemed to be part of a predestined plan, unaccompanied by previously envisaged fear or hysteria. My main emotion was intense curiosity at finding myself the central figure in a familiar scene. Conversation with my anaesthetic colleague was cut a little short . . . the next memory was of a series of persons looking down and making remarks in very rapid succession that could not be recorded. Later, like reaching the calm of the river below after shooting the rapids, I awakened amazed to find myself intact, with a dull ache in the right hypochondrium. The miracle had happened, and now my own effort must begin.

The textbook description of the postoperative period following cholecystectomy needs great amplification. The period is divided into three stages:

1. The *bed-of-nails stage.* — This lasts two days, and pain seems to emanate from every sensory perceptor in the body. All power is removed from muscles both above and below the incision, leaving very little that can be actively contracted at will. In this stage the attendants can extract any sum of money or promise for the future in return for an Omnopon injection which is the only resort of the destitute.

2. The *stage of the rack* follows in the next two days. All four limbs become fixed in extension; the body gradually slips down the bed; and the spreadeagling becomes fixed by the pain and spasm in the wound. This can be overcome only by the nurses bending the body forwards beyond the point of critical flexion, despite all hysterical protests. Both these stages are dominated by the patient's struggles to cough without tearing open the incision which at each attempt seems inevitable. These struggles last throughout the day and night and result in the patient assuming most unnatural positions. This is a practical illustration of the effect of an upper abdominal incision

which seems to strike at the root of normal respiration.

3. The *knife-in-the-side stage.* — Suddenly the patient awakens on the fifth day and feels confident that he is going to survive, there having been some slight doubt until then. He can breathe and cough and is delighted to find his other physiological functions returning to normal. He is still affected by a continuous ache in the incision, but this is nuisance value only. He now goes for walks with his physiotherapist, who, however, will not accept his explanation that he can only *either* straighten his knees *or* hold his head back on walking, but demands both. The removal of drain and sutures at this stage is like whistling in the wind by comparison with his previous troubles — pleasant distractions in the daily routine. He now feels up to taking a final-year group through the postoperative management of cholecystectomy. His confidence is returning; during the first two stages he made a final vow never to submit any human being to a major abdominal operation, but he is now coming round to the view that everyone should have a cholecystectomy.

With no interesting complications, I went home on the twelfth day, rather to the apprehension of my family. This is the time for philosophical reflection. What has been gained from the experience? First, a tardy and reluctant agreement with my wife's axiom that every abdominal surgeon should have had an abdominal operation; then, the equally reluctant recognition that no single person is indispensable in surgery, and that operations can be done equally successfully by others. This leads on to the reminder that surgery today is a team effort, and I am profoundly thankful to have been able to place my confidence in a team of like-minded colleagues. Finally, a shared experience with my patients will inevitably produce greater understanding.

# Chapter IX

# Coeliac Disease

Like so many patients with adult coeliac disease, my disorder
was not fully manifest or diagnosed until late middle life. But
there is every reason to believe that the gluten intolerance, which
is the chief characteristic of the declared disease, arises much
earlier in life. In describing the nature and effects of adult
coeliac disease I shall comment upon three phases, in childhood,
in adult life before diagnosis, and finally at the time when the
disease is fully evident. In retrospection it is all too easy to
sweep every vagary of behaviour into one obsessive net, and I
have been scrupulous to avoid this. Nevertheless, this account
is personal. The effects of disordered physiology on any human
being must be described through images particular to that person,
and any description of symptoms is so subjective that it would
vary greatly even if patients were trying to convey exactly the
same experiences, whereas the clinical range of coeliac disease
is considerable. Therefore I will emphasise that this is my account
and not necessarily the next fellow's, though I would hope that
there is sufficient common ground for him repeatedly to say,
"yes, I recognize that".

It was when I was about four years old that my parents seem
to have had misgivings about my health. I was examined by
doctors and stool specimens were taken and I was for a time
given a special diet, which consisted, interestingly, of the sub-
stitution of malted bread for the ordinary kind. Soon after this
my family went for a year to Africa, where I arrived with
paratyphoid fever, contracted on shipboard, severe enough to
render me unconscious, but afterwards health anxieties seem to
have faded, and both the tropical sojourn and the resumption of
life in Britain were uneventfully achieved. During school days I
developed a severe form of primary tuberculosis complicated by
pericarditis, of which the scars are very evident still. Any illness
was inclined to leave me wan for longer than other children, and
this, together with a terrible shyness, enveloped me in a cloak of
frailty which I turned to profit whenever possible, but which
was basically irksome to me. Coeliac children, deprived of the

48

irrepressible physical well-being that is the main-spring of adventurousness, are perhaps timorous by nature. During adolescence my puberty was somewhat delayed and during this long drawn-out process I underwent a remarkable growth spurt to reach a height of well over six feet, exceptional in my family, and certainly unusual in coeliac disease. One speculates whether delayed closure of the bony epiphyses allowed at this stage a longer than average growth stimulus to have a supernormal effect. Whatever the reason, I emerged as an elongated, rather tired-looking medical student, introspective and inhibited, but adept enough to qualify as a doctor before my twenty-second birthday.

My first experiences after qualification were in the Navy, and here I soon learnt something about alcohol. Although readier than most to welcome the loosening of inhibitions that it provided, nevertheless I found it treacherous to a degree quite out of proportion to its effects on my contemporaries, leading to a dyspepsia and prolonged loss of well-being if indulged in to the mildest excess. Likewise I found myself rather incapable as a smoker. Two days of sucking at a pipe or smoking cigars always led to a profound soreness of the tongue. But this conferred no immunity to cigarette addiction, and a twenty year struggle ensued to master this, not because of fears about ultimate effects so much as to the clear appreciation that a cigarette increased my nervousness and made it harder rather than easier to make social contacts. In spite of this, for many years I smoked about ten a day, perennially a victim to the perilous allure of the first cigarette of the day, and ensnared thereafter. The first puffs led to a gush of mildly vertiginous euphoria, followed quickly by an increase in nervous tension and a slight tremulousness of the limbs, symptoms perhaps of hypoglycaemia. As I got older these unpleasant physical side-effects became increasingly notable, and I felt less well when smoking, so that slowly I was able to master the habit.

Central to my life at this time, and indeed always, was the awareness of being somehow more than ordinarily enslaved by my body. Whereas the sensibility of most people seemed to rest like a cork on a full bottle of wine, close to but above the vital fluid, my own cork was pressed so far down that consciousness was constantly immersed in the bodily liquor, or so it seemed, and it was impossible by whatever effort of will to retreat from it. Accordingly, the physical effects of emotion, of fatigue, or of minor ailments were disproportionately intense. I came to associate this over-reactivity with my thinness, with the lean and hungry look, and when I compared myself, tense and interiorly occupied in maintaining an outward semblance of calm, with my friend, calm with the effortless naturalness of the normal, I cast covetous looks at his rounded limbs and plumper cheeks, and saw in a coating of adipose tissue possible rescue from an almost intolerable state. Later, one of the best effects of a gluten-free diet was to procure this rescue; to provide together with the long-sought extra layer of fat, a new inner sense of security and self-mastery. Battling all my life with this pathological hypersensitivity has squandered to no purpose a very great deal of mental energy. I discovered that so-called tranquillisers were very helpful to me in tiding over difficult ordeals, and indeed absolutely necessary on important occasions if I was not to give an account of myself ludicrously unrepresentative of my ability. At this time I would resort to phenobarbitone, and later to librium, with very ambivalent feelings towards their use, upbraiding myself for finding them necessary, and being conscious of a dimming of brightness and sparkle when sedated. But it is undoubtedly true that to the extra self-command so provided I owe a number of the minor achievements of my life.

At about thirty my hair started to turn grey, and by the early forties I was wholly grey, in contrast with what has happened to other members of my family. This is another coeliac symptom, but I then paid it no more than rueful attention as perhaps another tiresome by-product of a worrying nature.

I have always been unable to do without sleep. As I got older I became even more sleep-dependent, and would look unduly tired and shadowed if I didn't get enough. After a longish stint of work I quickly became grey and drawn, and was accustomed to being told "how tired you look", while never able to parry a resulting wave of depression. Once at an interview my appearance was such that the experienced physician in whose presence I was, remarked "you look ill: too tired. You should get yourself medically overhauled." But I *knew* that I was not ill, for I had no symptoms and enjoyed life, and was sure that a holiday would soon make me look better. And indeed it invariably did. Within hours of setting out on holiday my appearance changed. A healthy glow would appear on my blanched cheeks, and although there was seldom much change in weight, the effect of holidays in re-establishing my dormant vitality was apparent to all. This dependence of physical well-being upon freedom from workaday worries is exaggerated in chronic diseases, and the pale cast of thought seems to deepen their inroads upon the constitution. Not that my work was truly worrying. By this time I had taken up my chosen specialty and was happy in it. My work was not exacting. In fact, the discrepancy between my fatigued exterior and my inner conviction of health and competence, caused me much discouragement. For most of the time I truly felt well, and looking back with after-knowledge for disregarded symptoms there is still little to retrieve, unless perhaps the fixity of body weight at about one and a half stones less than the average for my height. But I had no digestive symptoms, or perhaps just one, and this one not available for comment, and indeed not so much a symptom as a curiosity, namely the fact that my stools and flatus have possessed from childhood a different and distinctive odour, something that had been remarked upon at school (where such matters are discussed) and had persisted since. It was to disappear finally when a gluten-free diet was started. Something else relevant was that during tropical service in the war, the intestinal upsets that are the lot of all, were for me more intense and longer lasting. Indeed after two years in the tropics I was seldom free from mild diarrhoea, and experienced a distressing prostration. I have also been afflicted with more than the ordinary number of common colds, both at home and abroad, seeming to develop less immunity to them than do others. One is tempted, uncertainly, to link this with the disturbance in immunoglobulins known to be present in many patients with coeliac disease.

In my late twenties I married. While somewhat less of a sexual athlete than many young men, after some initial difficulties I believe that this aspect of my life has always been fairly normal. Whether the long gaps between our three children indicate some degree of male infertility in the partnership can only be speculative.

In the lives of everyone there are probably moments when bubbles of joy rise unbidden into consciousness from some interior reservoir, and fill one briefly with unexpected happiness. Sometime in my middle forties this fortifying effervescence ceased. I thought that this was because I was getting older. At about the same time too I found myself more tired in the evenings after work. It was no longer possible to consider a social engagement on top of a day's work, and though in truth I was working harder, and accepted this as the explanation, the degree of fatigue was excessive. It would come over me like a narcotic soon after the evening meal and frequently I would retire to bed by 10 p.m. or earlier. On the other hand, I found it no longer possible to sleep on in the mornings and would wake early with ill-defined abdominal discomfort, and lie restless till the morning. If, on the evening before, I had had any alcohol, even a glass of wine, the abdominal discomfort and sleeplessness were greatly aggravated. I began, too, to have bad days. I would awake tired and headachey, without the normal amount of "go", and such days were dragged through with little enjoyment, longing for the relaxation of the evening. I was conscious at such times of a cold, blood-drained state of face and extremities, the very contrary of a healthy glow, and of a tired feeling around the eyes, fully corroborated by the mirror. Such days came more and more frequently (I regarded them as migraine), but on the others life was still normal and even exhilarating. But by the time holidays came I was seriously in need of them, but for the first time in my life the ebullient restoration conferred by holidays was absent. Even on holiday, grey days of physical depression made their appearance, and two weeks break would still find me unready to resume. Gradually, too, I was becoming a little disordered in digestion, with loss of appetite, rather faddy, and with a permanent and increasing "windiness" which was an embarrassment. Bowel habit was little altered, though at times there was a tendency to softness and looseness, especially when under mental pressure, though never to frequency of stools. I began to find the day-to-day perturbations of work difficult to deal with, to worry unduly about future happenings that might prove taxing, and to try to husband my energies. Towards afternoon I would be aware of a disagreeable nervous tension seeming to have its centre in the lower abdomen, which always presaged irritability and desperate fatigue at the end of the day.

Nevertheless, I was still quite without suspicion that there was anything physically wrong with me. All these symptoms I privately ascribed to psycho-neurosis. Contemptuous of such manifest constitutional inadequacy, I sought despairingly to battle with and conquer these derisory physical expressions of basic character weakness. Realisation that there was also a physical contribution did not dawn until about eighteen months after my mouth had become sore. One summer when I was 48 I experienced for the first time, after a severe cold, a general reddening and soreness of the mucous membrane of the tongue and cheeks. It lasted for some weeks, and recurred at intervals afterwards, especially over the tip and sides of the tongue, and inner surfaces of the lips. Eventually, after many months the true explanation for this, namely folic acid deficiency, dawned on me and a series of diagnostic investigations established at last, at the age of 49, that I had coeliac disease.

By this time I had lost a little weight and was generally considered to be cadaverously thin. A tiresome new symptom of
abdominal pain, a sort of central ill-defined gut-ache, had now
appeared and would wake me at night and lead to further sleeplessness. This was experienced only at night, and was quickly
abolished by standing upright. Another embarrassing symptom
was the persistent tendency of my stools to float. This I had
noticed from time to time throughout my life, but latterly this
had reached a point where it was difficult to flush them away,
and I was constrained on occasion to enervating sessions of plug-
pulling as a consequence. But the event that precipitated diagnosis
was a quite intractable period of mild diarrhoea after a summer
gastro-enteritis contracted in Ireland, which just would not end.

I'was rightly considered to be a mild case of coeliac disease,
and so the first treatment consisted only of a daily dose of folic
acid. This I continued for about a year. There were no further
attacks of severe soreness of the mouth, though even this
symptom was not entirely abolished, but when the mild euphoria
springing from a physical diagnosis and a treatment had worn off,
there was little other discernible effect. In fact things gradually
got rather worse, so much so that on one or two occasions when
at a low ebb I tried a small (5 mgm) dose of prednisone. The
effect was striking. Twenty-four hours after the dose I felt
entirely different, lost all my abdominal discomfort, and was
aware of a resurgence of energy and optimism. At the same time
my stools became firmer and darker. The effect was brief, not
outlasting twenty-four hours, and there were troublesome side-
effects from the drug, overaction of the heart, shortness of
breath and total insomnia, which combined with a healthy
awareness of the perils of steroid treatment to determine me
each time to keep the experiment brief. But it did allow me to
realise that a return to a state of well-being was not impossible.
It was this realisation which decided me eventually to accept
the difficulties and disadvantages for my family of a gluten-free
diet, and to embark upon it. In the event these difficulties were
largely illusory. My wife took a constructive attitude to the diet
from the beginning and is an excellent cook so that very soon
she became interested in exploding the shibboleths that have
arisen around the diet; that one cannot make certain articles such
as pastry, spaghetti, cake and so on, from gluten-free flour. Each
problem was attacked and vanquished, and I now have very few
dietary exclusions at home.

Within a few days of starting a gluten-free diet I became
aware of an extraordinary change. I was conscious of a warm

glow in my skin, and the pallid greyness of a few years past was replaced by a warm pink complexion. A similar metamorphosis was taking place within. I soon felt more self-confident, optimistic and energetic. I had no longer the same need to spare my energies; I could work hard all day and still have reserves. Meanwhile my appetite increased and my weight which had been fixed at 10¾ stone all my life (until recently when it had fallen lower), steadily rose, until after six months on the diet it was 13 stones. There it had remained ever since with the same unfluctuating constancy as formerly it showed at the lower level. The effect of steroids on my stools was reproduced by gluten elimination; not only did they become darker but also quite soon they no longer floated. Perhaps the happiest result was the rediscovery of joie-de-vivre, and of unsuspected stores of calm and stability to draw upon. Many of what I had taken for neurotic reactions proved to have been founded on bodily derangement, though patterns of behaviour consequently established were by this time more or less ineradicable.

There was therefore a most remarkable regenerative effect from the removal of gluten from my diet, and this has persisted through the three years that I have now been without it. But though life-transforming, it is not a cure; certain symptoms remain. During the first year of the new regime relapses occurred fairly frequently. I would wake with the "gluten feeling", a chill sense of abdominal unease and the pervasion of some deadly ichor throughout my body. The old fatigue would be there again, with a feeling of abdominal distension, mild constipation and a return of pallor and floating of the stools. After a few days such episodes would end. They were nearly always accompanied, and sometimes preceded, by a mild soreness of the mouth and tongue, and this last symptom has never been absent for more than a few weeks together, although true relapses have become very much less frequent. Efforts to attribute relapses to dietary transgression have not been successful, and it seems that nervous influences such as a period of hard work with loss of sleep, or demanding social functions, are more likely to produce them. But often no cause can be assigned.

Furthermore, I have become increasingly intolerant of even small amounts of alcohol, and have had reluctantly to abandon an evening aperitif because of the likelihood of a bad night afterwards. This alcohol-sensitivity increases during the day. At lunch I can usually tolerate a glass of wine without disturbance. I have noticed, too, a cushioning effect to the effects of alcohol from librium. I have taken this tranquilliser only seldom in the past few years, but under its influence seem able to drink a normal amount without after-effects.

This, then, ends my chronicle up to the present, and I have written it at such length because this disorder must be recognised as life-long, and to illustrate how easily its disguises can be misinterpreted, and the diagnosis overlooked, even by a doctor working amongst doctors.

My earliest memory is of being sick into my platter when bread and milk was presented to me, when oatmeal porridge ran out of stock. I did this four times when made to eat it again, and each time was spanked by our stern Victorian nurse with a toy cricket bat. At last I kept it down long enough to get to the garden and presented it at last as a "gift to the birds". Always detesting bread and cake, I loved potato and the garden roots and fruits, and could deal well with fish and meats.

But starvation, or else some bread, was at times the only alternative, and each time even the stalest bread sooner or later gave me trouble. I suffered from "growing pains" and "scleritis" of the eyeball, once with corneal ulcers and hypopyon; and from tenosynovitis of forearm muscle-sheaths. Eventually army biscuit and French bread, our only carbohydrate in France, caused, by winter 1915-16, such huge bursae under both Achilles tendons that I could only shuffle about in heelless slippers. This made my C.O. transfer me to the Australian Army Medical Corps from his R.A.M.C. unit. The voyage with Gallipoli convalescents enabled me to avoid gluten, and in Melbourne, part-military and part-civilian practice kept me well. In 1923 slowly progressive multiple sclerosis made me sell out and come to England, to consult Sir James Purves-Stewart who claimed to be able to cure or greatly improve M.S. The voyage made me so sea-sick from vertigo and ataxic nystagmus that I soon found that only arrowroot, rice, sago, mashed potato and fruit would stay down. On arrival, I found that the Harley Street doctors, even the famous surgeon Cecil Joll, were keen on the diet that Sir James said was his cure, Metchnikoff's "Balkan" diet of rough oats (kibbled as it was then called). He told me that I was by then in good remission and should remain so. I did not then recognise how important potassium was to prevent anxiety and depression, for lately it has been found that intra-cellular potassium was always very low in the brains of depressed suicidal patients.

So I still regarded myself as "damaged goods" and when doing a "locum" in a death vacancy, I boarded with a very determined widow, who demanded that I eat her excellent

pastry and pies etc. Then a bad state of depression set in. Only
after securing a happy marriage with an adaptable and obedient
wife, did I manage to revert to my gluten-free diet.

But the damage to my bones had been done, and in 1955 an
"intercostal neuralgia", suspected to be cholecystitis, led to
several X-ray examinations. These showed my vertebrae to be
porous, and collapsed into wedges, with Schmorl's nodes, and
links that led the radiologist to a diagnosis of ankylosing
spondylitis and spondylolysthesis. The spinal column pointed
straight down into the pelvic basin.

Then I started Calciferol Co. tablets, and as my life-long
steatorrhoea began to alternate with bouts of constipation I
luckily started magnesium sulphate at intervals of three or
four days. The X-rays of 1955 showed the usual coeliac distension of both small and large guts and colonic diverticulosis; so
to avoid the possible diverticulitis, I again reverted to black rice
and more regular Mist alba.

In 1968, 10 days after eating politely a big slice of birthday
cake on my 80th birthday a disc prolapse of L4–5–S1, and
increased angulation at L5–S1, caused a paraplegia which
extended from the hip area downwards. Three weeks of leg and
later pelvic-band traction, relieved me enough to walk with a
Zimmer frame, and to walk for about a mile.

Whether the haemolysis and fibrolysis which I believe afflicts
me when I take salicylates, sulphonamides and ampicillin is a
usual accompaniment in some cases of coeliac disease I am not
sure. Perhaps it might be lack of G6PD as recorded in 20% of
male W. African negroes. Dr. Badenoch mentions easy haemolysis in some of his cases. At least it has saved me from stiffness of
all my joints; even my right knee gave me no trouble for twenty-
five years after I was shot accidentally by a Home Guard in the
right popliteal space. The shot was lodged in the cartilage of the
origin of a crucial ligament of that joint. It suddenly disappeared
and went to my left lung, when I was in hospital for traction
for the paraplegia. After three weeks I could return home, with
a Zimmer walking aid and sticks.

The main lesson to be learned from my life-long illness is that
a multiplicity of illnesses, apparently disconnected, may arise
from a single cause, intestinal malabsorption due to gluten
sensitivity.

Chapter X

# Compression Fracture of Lumbar Spine

From October 1947 to March 1951, I was employed as a senior Army Pathologist at Fayid on the Suez Canal. I had had two previous tours abroad. The first was in India from 1934 to 1939, the the second in Egypt, Iraq, Palestine, Persia, and the north-east frontier of India from 1941 to 1945. I arrived back in England in March 1951. In June 1951, I had a slight fall from a stationary bicycle. I landed hard on my buttocks and sustained a compression fracture of the 12th thoracic vertebra. The X-ray also showed osteoporosis.

The pain was excruciating. However, I was just able to move and with the assistance of two workmen was moved upstairs to my own bed. From there I was taken to the local hospital. The next day I was moved by ambulance to Queen Alexandra's Military Hospital, Millbank, where I spent the next six weeks.

When the senior orthopaedic surgeon came to see me two days later, he told me to turn over in bed. I did so by grasping the side of the bed and pulling myself over with my arms. My legs were almost useless. For about three weeks I lay on my back day and night with a small firm pillow under the site of fracture. It was painful to turn on my side. If I tried to do so in my sleep, the pain at once woke me up. After about three weeks I started extension exercises under the instruction of the physiotherapist. At the end of July, I went to the Officers' Convalescent Home at Osborne for a month, where the exercises were gradually increased. By the end of September I was again fit for duty.

At Millbank I was looked after adequately but unimaginatively, I was in a room by myself. It was newly painted with a shiny white ceiling and no curtains over the two big windows. Consequently I was woken daily at 4 a.m. by the summer sun, until my wife came and fitted some curtains which she brought from home. The best the Army could do was to let me have a red bedpan screen! As I was mildly concussed from the fall, headaches were quite unpleasant until I could get some rest from the light. I lay flat on my back. My meals were placed on a bed table above eye level. At every single meal I was given a knife and fork. At every single meal I had to ask for a spoon, because I was unable to eat with a knife and fork without dropping food over myself and the sheet and pillow. In my helpless state, I found this unnecessary irritation upsetting to my temper.

There was quite a pleasant picture over the mantelpiece at the foot of my bed. After a couple of weeks, I asked if it would be possible to change it. I was told that it was a Red Cross arrangement and could not be altered. As I could see nothing from my bed except a few chimneys and the smoke of the steam trains entering and leaving Waterloo Station, I longed for something fresh to look at. When at last I could get up, I changed the picture with one from the next room. No one said anything. However, the Red Cross were able to lend me a portable radio set and there was a good Red Cross library service. I was also able to sew some tapestry chair seats, each of 40,000 stitches, which we still use in our dining room, so that my time was not completely wasted. My family and friends too were wonderfully good about coming to visit me.

When I was convalescent, I was fitted with a linen belt, which extended from the xiphisternum to the symphysis pubis. In front, it has five buckles and canvas straps. At the back, there are four thicknesses of cloth. Incorporated into it is an inverted V of half inch steel, 11½ in. (29 cm) long, which exactly fits the curve of my spine. I still use it whenever I get any serious pain in my back. The firm immobilisation given by the steel strip at the back, and the five straps in front alleviates the pain at once.

How could it happen that at the age of 42 I had senile osteoporosis of the spine? In the winter of 1936-7, while spending three months in the south of India, I had immense fatty frothy "sprue" stools. These were apparently due to the low protein diet, and cleared up soon after I got back to the north of India and normal army rations again. As I had had no serious diarrhoea for 15 years, not even in the Middle East and India during the war, I do not think that steatorrhoea had anything to do with it's causation. What is far more likely is that during my 3½ years in Egypt, practically my only exercise was swimming in the Great Bitter Lake. It kept me fit, but my back received none of the slight jolts with it gets as one walks. My blood urea was also slightly above normal at Millbank, but it has never been above 57 mg% and causes no symptoms. I am not hypertensive.

That however, was neither the beginning nor the end of my back troubles. I had been a wicket keeper throughout my cricket career and started to play again when I went to Egypt in 1947.

I had two crippling attacks of lumbago within a few months of one another, and so decided that my cricketing days were over. Unfortunately that did not stop the attacks of lumbago and sometimes of generalised "fibrositis". These would come on after quite mild physical exercise, such as trimming a garden hedge or jacking up the wheel of the car. I could usually manage to continue at work by using my belt to immobilise my lower back, but once or twice I had to go to bed for a few days.

In 1965, two things happened. I had a fall on the slippery floor of a shop, which jarred both the hip, on which I fell, and also the site of the old fracture. I strapped myself into my belt and was able to carry on with my work. For a few days I wore the belt day and night. After that, I had to travel about a hundred miles by car. At the beginning of the journey I was stiff and in pain. As the journey continued, the pain got less, and in a few days I was almost back to normal. The other factor was that I got a new firm mattress for my bed, a Slumberland Amber. Since I have used that, and since I have avoided working for more than a few minutes at a time with a bent back, I have been almost free from pain. I am always careful to lift anything heavy by bending my knees and keeping my back straight. An exercise which I occasionally use if my back gets painful is to hang with arms outstretched from the banisters or the top of a door with my feet off the floor. I do this for about a minute. It eases the pain surprisingly quickly.

Twenty years after the accident, I can still touch my feet without bending my knees, and can run and walk as far as most sixty year olds. Long may this happy state of affairs continue!

Chapter XI

# Coronary Disease

### John Hunter's Heart

John Hunter's fame made him the best known patient with angina. He wrote of it: "I was attacked suddenly with a pain nearly about the pylorus; it was a pain peculiar to those parts, and became so violent that I tried every position to relieve myself, but could get no ease. I then took a teaspoonful of tincture of rhubarb, with thirty drops of laudanum, but still found no relief. As I was walking about the room, I cast my eyes on a looking-glass, and observed my countenance pale, my lips white, and I had the appearance of a dead man looking at himself. This alarmed me. I could feel no pulse in either arm. The pain still continuing, I began to think it very serious. I found myself at times not breathing; and being afraid of death soon taking place if I did not breathe, I produced a voluntary action of breathing, working my lungs by the power of my will. I continued in this state three quarters of an hour, when the pain lessened, the pulse was felt, and involuntary breathing took place." His later death from coronary thrombosis occurred at St. George's Hospital when, "meeting with some things which irritated his mind and not being perfectly master of the circumstances he withheld his sentiments; in which state of restraint . . . he gave a deep groan and dropt down dead".

With a high familial rate of coronary heart disease, mostly on the maternal side, I had been cognisant for many years of the fads and fancies of the nutrition experts and epidemiologic-ally minded cardiologists. I had not taken sugar in drinks or on food for 25 years. I avoided carbohydrates and lived on pro-teins, vegetables, and fruit, my ration of flour being restricted to about 1 or 2 slices of bread daily. When it was suggested that animal fats were possibly atherogenic, butter was limited to a scrape occasionally, all food was grilled, fat was removed from meat and corn oil was substituted in salads and in cooking. For the last 20 years my alcohol intake consisted of about 1 to 2

pints of beer per week and 2 to 3 gins daily, with the odd party
once a week or fortnight. Cigarettes were eventually given up
4 years ago, but I smoked 1 to 2 ounces of tobacco weekly and
the occasional cigar. My work consisted of driving for 5 miles
to arrive at my consulting rooms at about 9 a.m., seeing perhaps
20 patients in a morning session until 11 or 11.30 a.m., then
doing a few house calls when I usually ran upstairs always
fighting against the clock, driving a nippy car in frustratingly
slow traffic, eager to be at the next place to do my job with as
little waste of time as possible: then back home across Bristol for
lunch at 1 p.m. which was probably completed by 1.15 p.m.
The afternoon was filled by dictating letters, seeing special
patients at home or doing clinics at hospitals. Tuesdays and
Thursdays were particularly long days. I have had no real
exercise since giving up rugger at 24 years, except for gardening
or doing general odd jobs about the house. I was, however, always
active and my weight, clothed, had been around 13 st. 3 lbs. ±
7 lbs. since 21 years. Apart from an appendicectomy, a hernia
repair and tonsillectomy, I had only had the odd day in bed for
minor complaints.

About 4 years ago, I woke up one night with a peculiar
sensation in my chest and a rapid and irregular pulse, which
lasted about 2 hours. From that time I have had similar attacks
at varying and irregular intervals. On one particular occasion I
was able to have an E.C.G. taken in an attack and this revealed
atrial fibrillation. Sent by my wife to see a cardiologist friend, I
was shaken to learn, after his very meticulous clinical examination,
E.C.G. and screening, that I had a slight aortic incompetence,
inverted T.V5 & 6 and B.P. $\frac{160}{100}$. My immediate reaction was to
rush home and take my own blood for serology. Although I had
never had any symptoms or signs, I was relieved when the results
were returned as normal as was my serum cholesterol and blood
culture. These attacks did not really worry me and only occured
after working or playing too hard.

On Saturday, 8th November, a week before my 61st birthday,
I had not had an attack of atrial fibrillation for about 6 months
and I had not been exerting myself unduly. I did routine work
on the Saturday forenoon, rushed across Bristol to see a patient
at home and then entertained a nephew and his new wife for the
weekend. We motored down to Wells and after driving round and
round to find a park, walked round the old town and cathedral.
In the evening, before dinner, I had 2 gins, wine with dinner and
a whisky later and smoked 2 cigars. Before retiring about 12 p.m.
I was conscious of slight central chest discomfort. I locked up

the house and went to bed, falling asleep almost at once. At 2 a.m. I awoke with an unpleasant sensation in the centre of my sternum and recognised immediately what had happened, because I also had an uncomfortable feeling in my right elbow. Not wishing to disturb my wife, I lay awake, restless with this discomfort. One certainly could not describe it as a pain, but it was sufficiently disturbing to prohibit sound sleep. By 8 a.m. I had no symptoms at all. However, I rang up a physician friend who examined me and did an E.C.G. confirming an anterior infarction. I remained in bed without any symptoms and on Monday evening began searching through the contents of my safe, brought to me by my wife, for insurance policies, and became rather frustrated by not finding one which later I realised had been terminated at 60 years. I settled down for sleep at 10 p.m. with 200 mg Tuinal, but awoke at 2 a.m. with a different, unpleasant hard central chest pain with again associated discomfort in my right elbow. Rate and rhythm were normal. Foolishly I had no analgesics in my room, so I took 400 mg Tuinal at 2 a.m. and on 2 further occasions during the night, but had no sleep. On Tuesday morning my physician friend gave me 10 mg of morphia and sent for the ambulance to take me to the Bristol Royal Infirmary. I vaguely remember being lifted out of bed into a chair for transport and later waking, propped up in a hospital bed with 3 electrodes on my left chest connecting me to the monitor. I had no further chest pain while in hospital for 12 days and none since, but for six weeks I was aware of the left side of my chest, particularly if lying on that side or when walking about.

After 4½ weeks, when my routine was to get up at 11 a.m., sleep for 2 hours after lunch and then retire about 10 p.m., I went to sleep at 10.30 p.m. and awoke at 2 a.m., conscious of an odd discomfort in my chest and a rapid irregular pulse of about 90 per minute. Later in the night I was disturbed again by a change of rhythm — apparently regular tachycardia of 120 per minute. Later, toward morning, this changed to irregular rhythm of 90 per minute again. After a warm bath for 10 minutes, I reverted unconsciously to normal rhythm at 80 per minute. After that I was digitalised and since the 7th week, have not been conscious of any further sensation in my left chest. Apart from some feebleness on walking, I am no different from before 8th November and have no angina or dyspnoea.

In 1927 my father stimulated my interest in Samuel Pepys. Since that time I have kept a reasonably full personal diary, from which an account of the following events is derived.

The year 1947-1948 proved to be unusually hectic. Having been invited by the Honorary Staff of my hospital to develop haematology, a postgraduate award facilitated visits to Oxford, London, Edinburgh and Glasgow in rapid succession and for varying periods of time. I returned, on the 16th March, 1948, when I was aged 30 years. While holding a tutorial for conjoint students four symptoms occurred in rapid succession and within seconds of each other. Initially the undergraduates and their surroundings became blurred. Then a feeling as though a heavy weight was pressing on the lower sternum was followed by fluttering in the chest and then dyspnoea; the pulse rate was 120 per minute with many extrasystoles. At the same time I noted that the lower substernal pain was increased by pressure or tapping of this area. The pain (which has never recurred), feeling of faintness, fluttering and dyspnoea lasted for about 30 minutes. An E.C.G. was taken about 45 minutes after the onset. At this juncture I felt sufficiently well to telephone my wife, after which I was admitted to a ward and sedated.

After the next 48 hours, during which I slept most of the time, it became apparent that my physician had arranged for serial E.C.G.s and daily white cell counts and E.S.R. I was always grateful when an experienced laboratory technician came to perform the venepuncture! During the next few days five patients died on "my" ward and on the 21st March a member of my staff was admitted to the same ward with bronchopneumonia, when I experienced a further attack of fluttering in the chest but no other symptoms.

After returning home on 27th March I had three attacks of tachycardia, each lasting for about 20 minutes, the last associated with quite severe dyspnoea. I was readmitted to hospital the same day and sedated with barbiturate. Gradual improvement with fewer attacks of tachycardia and increased exercise tolerance was followed by discharge home on 13th April. On the 20th of that month I noted discomfort in the right tonsillar region associated with frequent extrasystoles. Treatment with quinidine gr. 3 b.d. was begun and continued until 27th June. During this period a tonsillar abscess was drained and steady improvement occurred, resumption of normal duties taking place on 10th May. Since then there have been no cardiac symptoms apart from an occasional extrasystole such as anyone may experience.

I later found out that the original E.C.G. showed right bundle-branch block which has remained unchanged certainly until about one year ago when I had a medical examination for insurance purposes. There is no family history of heart disease and I have now become a first-class life insurance risk.

*One of the most puzzling cases that I have met with occurred in a doctor, an able man and a good observer. He wrote to me on June 22, 1914, the following account of himself:

"I am in my 56th year, and have always had extremely good health — practically no illnesses of any kind whatever. I led a strenuous life in my early days, with plenty of night work, but I have always enjoyed very good health.

"In the spring of 1905 I did not feel very well — rather a loss of energy and keenness about things, and I thought I would examine my urine. I found about 15 per cent of sugar in the urine, and from that day to this I have dieted with the object of reducing the sugar, and when I diet very carefully I can be without sugar, though my capacity for digesting starch is extremely small. One potato or one piece of bread will bring back the sugar at any time, though I can take any amount of sugar in the form of fruit such as strawberries without the sugar increasing. In spite of the glycosuria I have had the very best of health, and have been able to work and play pretty hard. In fact, the strain in my practice in the summer months is very great indeed, as I see on an average about thirty-five patients a day. I did this work extremely well last summer, and enjoyed my winters' leisure. I took fairly long walks almost every day, and did Muller's exercises systematically every morning, followed by my usual cold bath, which I never missed in my life.

"On the 6th day of May last I went to bed feeling as well as usual, and about 2 o'clock I woke up in a dreadful panic with most acute anginal pains. I was quite alone, as my wife happened to be away at the time. The pain ran down the inside of my arm to my fingers, and was really very intense, but my pulse was quite good all the time, and I had no breathlessness to speak of. At first I was frightened of dying at once, but that feeling soon passed off, and the only thing was the intense pain just over the sternum. I went to sleep after a time, and the next morning felt quite well, and for a week nothing happened except once

* From Sir James Mackenzie's classic work "Angina Pectoris".

or twice a little tightness over the sternum when walking. I consulted a doctor friend, who examined me carefully. He found the blood pressure about 156 mm Hg, the heart sounds perfectly normal, and he did not attach very great importance to the attack. On the 13th, that is exactly a week after the first attack, I got the pain again whilst sitting with two doctor friends. The pain was, as before, very intense, but was quickly removed by amyl nitrite, which I then had. I got home, went to sleep, and woke up again to the same condition of affairs. After this I kept very quiet until the Friday, when I went out for a drive in my car and got a bad attack in it. On Saturday a consulting physician came over to see me, and his opinion was that there was no suspicion of organic disease, but he advised getting up late, going to bed early, having tea very weak, stopping smoking and giving up the cold bath, and taking the principal meal in the middle of the day. As for drugs he gave me 15 grains bromide of ammonium to take twice daily. Since that time I have been getting up late and doing my work, and as soon as it was finished going back to bed again. I never have the least bother in seeing patients in the study, and all the attacks have been while I have been at rest.

"All went well until Friday last, when, after getting to bed about 9 o'clock, the pain began again, and continued at intervals until after 12. Amyl did not give relief nor did nitro-glycerine help much. The most comfortable position I could get in was to kneel on the floor and throw the whole weight of my body on the bed, face downwards. The attack went off about 12, and I went to sleep, and since then I have been perfectly well. My blood pressure has been frequently taken, and it has never been more than 156 mm Hg, and the vessels seem quite soft.

"I may add that I have been extremely temperate as regards alcohol all my life, never having taken any except some light wine with meals. As to smoking, I have enjoyed it in the winter months and I used to have about three ounces of tobacco a week, and in the summer about an ounce and a half.

I have never myself met anything exactly like this, and I wondered whether it was the effect of the long-continued glycosuria. I think it is a neurosis, but I do not know what is best to do. I must work, if possible, until the end of October, after which I can take as much rest as is necessary and do anything that is desired.

"As to family history, my father was a confirmed asthmatic but lived to 66. My mother enjoyed excellent health, and had a splendid constitution. My only brother died three years ago very suddenly, and was found to have an enlarged fatty heart, but he lived a very strenuous life, and was not careful with either smoking or alcohol.

"My weight when I got the first attack was 13 st. 11 lb. Under this partial rest cure I have increased to 14 st. 7 lb."

He wrote again on July 17:

"I have been keeping perfectly well until a few days ago, when I was seized by a sudden pain down in the chest, and more to the left than the previous pain. I recognised at once that it was of a different character. It was extremely severe, and I was compelled to go to bed. Nothing gave relief, not even the injection of a grain of morphine. A little relief was obtained by inhaling chloroform. After some hours the pain subsided, and I got up next day. The following night I was awakened at 2 a.m. with a stabbing pain in the chest and a good deal of breathlessness. I examined my chest and found the front of the heart full of pericardial friction sounds. This was confirmed by a doctor later in the day, who applied six leeches, which gave immediate relief. The temperature was slightly raised for a few days. The blood pressure, which had been usually 150 mm Hg, was 126."

He wrote on March 1, 1915, stating that in December he went to a sanatorium, where he was dieted and treated with great care, and he said that he had greatly improved in health. While undergoing treatment, on January 8, 1915, he had an attack of dyspnoea when out walking and had to be taken home, when he had an acute attack of oedema of the lungs. He wrote: "I got quite blue and cold, and an immense quantity of frothy mucus flowed from my nose and mouth, and I was taken home and put to bed, and had a nasty hacking cough for eight hours, which brought up all the mucus, and then I got rapidly well."

He had a similar attack on February 17.

The patient wrote asking me to make an appointment, and I gave an appointment for March 7, but he did not keep it, telegraphing to say that he was laid up with another attack of acute oedema of the lungs. He died in an attack of this oedema a fortnight later.

The idea of illness affects people differently. As doctors we have a close association with disease, and our knowledge will affect us individually according to our temperaments. A doctor's attitude to himself can vary from the extreme anxiety which made a retired doctor of my acquaintance order a complete series of X-rays for himself annually, to an attitude of "it can't happen to me" and to a disregard of any symptoms in one's self as imaginary and hypocondriacal.

I think that I tend to be of the latter class. Experience of patients has taught me that fear of illness causes just as much distress as the illness itself which may well be absent, so that it seems a waste of time to worry until one is certain. Looking back now, I can remember a very cold day in the early 1940's when I did have quite a sharp pain in my chest on physical exertion. It was a completely isolated incident. I had hurried through a hectic morning's work in order to go and try to get a brace of partridges for the pot, the plough was very heavy to walk over, and there was a biting wind with snow in it. I had nearly given up trying to find the covey which I knew lay there or thereabouts, when I managed to get a long shot at them as they flew away, and one came down wounded but ran on. My dog had recently been killed and I had not yet got another, so I had to run myself: the bird got up and flew again just at extreme range and once again I hit it but did not kill it so that it ran on again. People who shoot and who read this will appreciate the situation, and my determination to get that bird, which I eventually did. I was about 40 at the time, and thought what a fool I was but I did not in fact take any further notice of the pain which went off quite quickly.

I forgot all about it and then in 1960 I had another reminder. I do not keep a diary, but I got into the habit of writing down an occasional page about any particular event or thoughts which I thought were worth capturing, and I looked back and found this one dated 1st August 1960: "Bank Holiday Monday, a bathe in Richard's pool before breakfast; then I tried to photograph the horses. At once the sun dodged in and out of the clouds. When it was sunny they posed in front of the gasometer; when I did get them right and produced the camera, they decided at once it must be good to eat.

A drinks party here, then lunch, and the afternoon up at the site of the new house, weeding the future bed by the gate, and my wife planning the shrubs and trees. Hot and tired, there was the pool again — and then death just tapped me on the shoulder and for a minute I smelt his breath. I have met him so often as he comes closer and closer to my patients; he can be no stranger to a country doctor: but one tends to think always that one's own call is some time off yet. It may be, but today left me a reminder that like everyone else, I have to face it some day, and it may be sooner than I expected.

Does familiarity make death more fearful, like one poor old doctor whom I watched thirty years ago in mortal terror? Shall I do better than he, and even though afraid, at any rate help my family by the one thing I can do — show no sign. Can I, in fact, honestly feel that sleep is good after the long day: relief that we do not have to struggle on too long, thankfulness for so much fun and happiness. Old men can be depressing creatures: so isn't it better to leave a bit early when the party is in full swing?

Five years after that when I was 60, I was in my consulting room one evening with a full appointments list. It was about half past five and I saw that I still had another ten patients to see: I had had a hard day and a hard week and as a lady came in, a difficult argumentative type, dissatisfied with life and taking it out of her family and the doctor in an effort to come to terms with her personal difficulties, I thought to myself "now what is it exactly I am trying to do with this patient?" And the answer came back loud and clear "get rid of her as quickly as possible". I was brought up rather short, because I had always imagined that I was enjoying my work; and had indeed taught students that mankind is divided into two classes, the ones who do a job in order to earn their living, and who will switch at any moment to a higher paid job: and the ones who work at something which they would do in any case out of the sheer joy of it, and which incidentally brings them in a reasonable living. Unless the student felt he belonged to the latter class he had better switch to the City while there was time. By easing my work and eventually retiring from the National Health Service, I got back my pleasure in medicine and I had the chance to take a good deal more strenuous exercise, hunting, shooting (and by that I mean walking the hedges rather than standing in line), sailing and fishing: and I never remember getting any symptoms of precordial pain or undue breathlessness considering that I was by then well over 60. I am neither short nor fat, and have smoked only very moderately for several years, latterly a couple of cigars a day, so that the last thing I expected was to join the coronary club.

But on November 27th 1969 I had a fairly extensive myocardial infarction. I was in London, in the middle of a week of committee work with theatre and dinners at night. The attack came on in the early hours of Thursday morning when I woke up cold and sweating with intense pain in my lower jaw. I cannot remember any feeling in my chest apart possibly from a

little pressure, and certainly none in my arms: but I felt
extremely ill and faint, with a tendency to be sick. I took my
pulse and found that it was of very poor volume, and it was
very slow — I timed it with a wrist watch and made it between
36 and 38 per minute, so I correctly assumed that I had a
complete heart block, and that there was a myocardial lesion in
the area of the bundle of His. I sucked a T.N.T. tablet, because
I had had a similar mild occurrence once or twice in the past, at
the same time in the early morning: both times I got quite well
in a short time after sucking a T.N.T. tablet, getting up and
moving round and having a drink of hot water: but this time
the T.N.T. made me feel if anything worse. After half an hour
or so I awakened my wife, who promptly took over and
telephoned a doctor friend who was round in a few minutes. I
remember little after this because he gave me an injection of
pethidine and got an ambulance. I have a vague recollection of
extreme difficulty in extracting me from one of the back rooms
of the club in which I was staying, and of being put into the lift
and then taken out down the stairs because the chair would not
fit in. I remember the ride in the ambulance and a reception
party at St. George's Hospital, a trolley and a lift upstairs and
then bed with a row of white coats round me.

In an interval of clarity I heard one of these say "We're just
going to put in a pacemaker and you will feel much better". I
promptly replied that I didn't want it, whereupon he said "Well
of course if you don't want it we can't force you" and the white
coats faded away.

Looking back, I realise that my reason for such a stupid refusal
of treatment was my lack of up-to-date knowledge on pacemakers. I had one patient some years ago who had a permanent
pacemaker in position, which undoubtedly kept her going when
it worked, but there were desperate emergencies when she had
to be transferred back rapidly to London from 40 miles away
when the pacemaker got temperamental. This was the impression
that persisted in my mind, and I suppose I had the feeling that if
I couldn't exist without that particular aid then I would rather
not do so at all.

However all was well, because my blood pressure fell — I
heard some voice saying "Well I make it 70 with no diastolic",
and my heartbeat continued at well under 40. A white coat
assured me that the pacemaker was only a temporary measure, 2
or 3 days. I at once said "Do carry on and put the pacemaker
in" and the same white coat said "Well it won't be quite so
easy now as if we had done it in the first place". A further

injection, a dim memory of someone hitting my chest violently at intervals, and then suddenly I felt quite bright again, I could see the pacemaker ticking away, and the wire leading to my right arm in a splint (there had been a drip in my left one from the start) and of course E.C.G. wires on my chest and an oxygen mask so I felt like something from outer space.

My recovery was uneventful, apart from a toxic rash, thrush from cloxacillin and the refusal of my heart to go back into normal rhythm for rather longer a period than is usual.

I have been asked what were my reactions at finding myself in a monitoring ward (intensive care): was I frightened, did I think I was going to die, or did I feel confident because of the care that was being taken of me and so on?

In fact none of these questions occurred to me at all, and on looking back I think it seems that I rather arrogantly assumed that I would get better as a matter of course. The unit was noisy from its very nature, a new arrival meant that there was a great deal of technical work to do, and there was no apparent effort to reduce noise even in the small hours of the morning. Looking back from some time afterwards I am quite sure that I was unconsciously given a great feeling of confidence by the obvious technical efficiency of the unit.

I think that the two points worth noting about this episode are:

1. The intense pain in the lower jaw, with no related precordial pain or pain in the arm.

2. The lack of correct post-graduate knowledge about pacemakers. In my case this was because we have not yet got them in the local hospitals; they are still concentrated in the larger centres.


My partial gastrectomy was two days old, and at 3 o'clock in the afternoon I was feeling well, though irked by the nasal tube, much more unpleasant than the drip. Five minutes later I knew something was wrong; at first it was no more than a general malaise. Then gradually I became conscious of slight right-sided pain on breathing, worsening until it was obviously pleuritic. A few hours later I was painfully coughing up blood and by then breathlessness had also developed. Later came a new pain, cramp-like and unremitting, almost immobilising the right side of my trunk, and to which the continuing pleuritic pain was a bagatelle.

So I lay, sweating, frightened, and scarcely able to move, with morphia welcomed for its easing of my misery. The next morning the agonizing constant pain had abated, and thirty-six hours later the complication seemed to be resolving. On the fifth day came more pain with breathing, a fresh haemoptysis, and once more the awful steady pain. During the night my bowels were open and I shall always remember the pain forcing me to lie motionless, with the degradation I felt at being so helpless, having to leave all to the nurses. Once more there came morphia and slowly resolution of the symptoms and signs. Not until the nineteenth day did I have phlebitis in my right calf.

The cause of the constant ceaseless pain, far and away the worst I have ever had? I think it must have been reflex muscular spasm.

Then came convalescence, the anxiety that the chest X-rays showed too slow a resolution, the fear of bronchial carcinoma, and the kindly chest physician who said, and rightly, "You have only fear to fear". Since then there has been complete relief from duodenal symptoms and the greatest boon, the tranquil nights, no longer being woken by pain.

So followed six years of hard and long, yet happy, hours of work, until a Sunday summer's morning when I was writing at my desk and became aware of a slight soreness under the sternum, relieved for a minute by belching. But then it returned with greater severity, a soreness, or perhaps a "rawness" best describes it. I had little doubt it was cardiac pain, though I tried an antacid in unrealised hope. The pain continued and increased, and though it couldn't be called unbearable, the unrelieved constancy was its worst characteristic.

Five minutes after its onset came a sudden drenching sweat, and shortly afterwards our family doctor. Pethidine didn't help and once more I experienced the power and peace of morphia.

E.C.G. confirmation of a myocardial infarct followed and the journey to my own hospital, into my own medical ward and to the care of the nurses with whom I worked: I know now how fortunate my patients are, nursing-wise. I cannot really remember much pain after the first two hours, nor indeed any fresh symptoms save for tiredness for a few days. The monitoring didn't worry me, physically or mentally, nor did I want to see the tracing. I had no fear of complications save only of a further lung infarct, and remember at first being quite cheerful, and probably even euphoric. But, as I progressed in convalescence, so depression developed. I do not think this was due to fear of dying, but because I knew I must accept my colleague's advice, that I had drastically to curtail my way of life. Strange how having hours of leisure time for country walks, and reading the journals, brought frustration rather than pleasure. Another cause — though perhaps this was after all fear of dying — was the loss of the integrity of one's body: indeed of oneself. All doctors and probably most educated men who have had a "coronary", must feel like the inhabitants of a besieged city, who have repelled one attack but who know that the breach has not been fully repaired and that one day their city must fall; whereas most illnesses represent an attack repulsed, and followed by complete repair of the defences. I find this difficult to describe, but I know now that there is a great contrast in possessing a body which merely creaks with age but has shown no evidence of serious disease, and one that is for ever suspect. I believe now that in the past I have treated the physical aspect of coronary disease in my patients as well as I could, but that I should have given much more time to sustaining their morale and, too, to keeping the wife informed, upon whom so many patients lean. One other cause for melancholy; a nicotine addict giving up tobacco, thereby gaining unwanted weight despite foreknowledge, and afterwards a reducing diet!

Finally, and inexplicable to me, is the sweating. Most cases sweat at first, presumably a reflex to pain. But this propensity has continued, and beads of perspiration will still develop after only modest exertion or in a warm room, a thing that never happened before. Infarcts are unpleasant, but to me the pulmonary ones were much worse physically, the cardiac one infinitely worse on the mental plane.

It was Christmas eve 1965 and my wife and children had retired to bed. I was sitting in my drawing room with a glass of whisky in my hand looking forward to Christmas day when suddenly I experienced a monstrous and to me terrifying pain within my chest; my glass of whisky fell to the floor. This pain was short-lived, lasting for a few seconds I believe, although it seemed much longer. I sat still for about half-an-hour and I recall that I had what I later described as a feeling of tightness within and about my chest and a dull pain. I went to bed and during the early hours of the morning experienced two more minor earthquakes.

I took part in all the family activities on Christmas day feeling a little odd but not uncomfortable. I did not tell my wife or anyone else about the previous evening. Late on Boxing day I suffered another major earthquake and so told my wife that I did not feel well and was going to see my doctor next day instead of returning to work.

It transpired that my doctor was away in Ireland; I rang one of his partners and he was ski-ing in Switzerland. The third partner saw me, listened to my story, examined me with much care and much patience, but could not discover anything wrong with me. He told me he would like me to be X-rayed.

Two days later I presented myself before a very distinguished radiologist; his technician took a number of pictures; she asked me to wait until the plates were developed. The chief came back and asked me how I had come to his rooms. I told him by car and that my wife and family were waiting in it below. He asked "does your wife drive?". "Yes" I replied; "then she must drive you home. Then go straight to bed; I shall be in touch with your doctor who will see you to-night". He accompanied me to the door, put his hand on my shoulder and told me to take things very quietly. I thanked him and then drove the family home. Later that evening my family doctor arrived with a portable electrocardiograph; the electrocardiograms he told me, and he showed them to me, were normal. He told me that my plates were to be sent to a cardiologist; meanwhile I was to stay in bed.

The following evening my wife, my brother and sister-in-law were with me when I felt another minor tremor and this time the left side of my body seemed to me to be both cold and clammy, the other side normal. I said to my sister-in-law "am I imagining things or is my body colder on one side?" She explored and said "how very odd, yes it is". I also had a warm metalic taste in my mouth. Later that night the doctor came and told me that I should have to go to a heart hospital as soon as it could be arranged. When we were alone I asked why and the words cardiac aneurysm were mentioned.

My wife told me later that she was given what, for her, must have been frightening instructions should certain things happen to me during the night. It was revealed 48 hours later that no beds were available and that the chosen cardiologist who had seen my X-rays had departed to Austria for a fortnight.

The next morning I decided to telephone a friend who is a consultant physician. Within hours I was in bed in one of the major teaching hospitals. I was in a cardiac ward and that evening was given sleeping drugs but about 2 a.m. I was awakened by another earthquake and in considerable pain. The ward was dimly lighted, quiet but for the sounds of snoring, and still except for the heart machines blipping away their regular, irregular and macabre messages. When sister appeared and asked why I was not sleeping I told her I was in some pain and asked for another pill; she explained that I had had my quota. Near to dawn the pain having subsided I slept only to be awakened and told to clean my teeth, which I was unable to do as these had been blown out during the battle of Caen in 1944.

For two days I told and re-told my experiences to a number of physicians. Numerous tests were carried out, new X-rays, new electrocardiograms were taken, blood and urine tests, a barium meal that I loathed, the soles of my feet were teased with cotton wool and pins stuck into me and rubbed down my spine. I was given a lumbar puncture — my only comment about the lumbar puncture that I wish to make is that I felt nothing but became bored at gazing at the ceiling for twenty-four hours.

The ward round started about 11 a.m. and the Senior Physician sat at the side of my bed and told me in friendly and gentle tones that there was nothing wrong with me and that the pain I had endured was known as root pain and he gave me a most lucid explanation of how this occurs. I was home next day, feeling a bit of a cheat. I have had no pain since.

Chapter XII

# Cranial Arteritis

While on vacation from locum work one Sunday morning, in late November 1969, my wife and I were sitting in our car parked on the sea front watching the tide come in when I noticed some symptoms which my wife thought were due to the onset of a cold. I told her that they were·not my usual symptoms.

The symptoms were post-nasal obstruction on the right side and pain in the soft tissues of the neck when swallowing. This pain was localised to very small areas, the size of a pinshead on all sides of the neck. The post-nasal obstruction was mild and the mucus was clear.

An E.N.T. surgeon examined me a few days later and found a deviated septum on the right side, with signs of acute. inflammatory changes localised to this side. An X-ray examination showed the sinuses were clear. The neck pain lasted for two days.

After this onset I developed, the next day, a right-sided headache. It came on in attacks, about three in the first 24 hours but after a few days more frequently, about three-hourly. It was a tense dull ache and was centred deep in the right side of the face. It appeared to start at the base of the skull where it was most intense and then spread from this small area to all over the right side of the head. Between these attacks there was a mild constant headache. On one occasion I was awakened with most severe headache and a sensation of the right side of the skull being distended considerably, this unpleasant condition lasting a few minutes.

This headache was associated with stabbing or shooting pain beginning in the right occipital region of the skull and then after two days in the pre-auricular region, the stabbing directed downwards and upwards, sometimes straight across the face or around the right auricle, right temporal region and right posterior palate, the intensity of the stabs increased as the acute condition developed. There was also tenderness along the upper aspect of the right zygoma, the lower border of the right mandible, over the greater cornu of the hyoid bone and over the supra-orbital and infra-orbital foramina.

Similar symptoms of headache and stabbing pain and tenderness affected the left side 14 days after the beginning of this illness; they were much less severe and lasted only a few days. Intermittent claudication of the temporal muscles was noticed on mastication, mainly at breakfast; this persisted for six weeks.

Visual changes occurred during the attacks of headaches and stabbing pain; they were:—

1. On the right side an appearance of a rectangular crown with flames coming from the apices.

2. On the right side an occasional appearance of a small circle, beautifully coloured, red, green, black and white.

3. For a few days an orange ball was seen behind and slightly above a nurses's ear when one was in the room.

4. Vision, at about 100 yards, became slightly indefinite.

5. Vision was blurred at times during the acute phase.

6. On one occasion a queer sensation of a snake orbiting the right eyeball; this was not painful but most alarming.

7. During an attack and almost all the time during the acute phase a bruised sensation in my eyelids when the eyelids were opened, so I had to keep my eyelids closed to relieve this; the eyeballs felt tired.

8. There was a sensation when the eyes were opened of a bar going midway across the right eyeball.

9. No photophobia at any stage, even on ophthalmic examination.

Vomiting developed after a few days and was associated with the attacks of pain; it was aggravated by oral therapy. I was not able to take aspirin or any tablet containing aspirin because it produced a few hours later excessive salivation, the saliva pouring from the salivary ducts — so fast that it was difficult to swallow it quickly enough. Tenderness of the temporal and occipital arteries began on the right side 12 days after onset and on the left side one week later. For three weeks taste was altered especially for tea and coffee, both being most unpleasant.

Biopsy of a portion of the right temporal artery confirmed the diagnosis of arteritis.

### Treatment

Within 48 hours of commencing prednisolone — 80 mg daily — the attacks became less severe and less frequent and after twelve days the attacks of headache and pain ceased. Prednisolone was reduced to 40 mg daily eight days after commencement, then to

30 mg daily two weeks later and 20 mg daily six weeks later, 15 mg daily two months later then 10 mg daily which is being continued.

Before steroid therapy partial relief was obtained at first by taking Panadol and then Fortral injections.

The complications, as a result of the arteritis or steroid therapy have been:—

1. Acute simple glaucoma — coming on two months after onset and giving rise to myopia. The glaucoma has responded to pilocarpine — 2% — eye drops. The myopia is controlled with lenses.

2. Tendonitis involving the right and left achilles tendons developed five months after onset and was localised to a small area of the tendons about two inches from their insertions into the os calcis. This complication caused very limited and painful walking which lasted two months but I had no pain or difficulty when driving a car.

3. General muscular weakness and some wasting in muscles of lower limbs, coming on about 5½ months after onset. It lasted two months. An electromyogram showed changes in some muscle groups of the left lower limb.

4. Symptoms suggestive of duodenal ulcer coming on two months after onset and lasting about four weeks. They responded to diet and alkalies.

5. General increase in subcutaneous tissue — especially in face and fingers, and more rapid growth of hair and nails.

## Chapter XIII

# Depression

In March 1954 I developed a persistent frontal headache. It was bilateral and rather above the area associated at times previously with mild migraine or frontal sinus infection. It came on after getting up and became worse as the day went on. I had a temperature just above normal on some evenings. This headache persisted for 3-4 weeks; then, one evening, just as I was going to bed, it suddenly "switched off", to be replaced by palpitation, sweating of the hands and feet, and a feeling of panic. I rang up my doctor, who told me to take two grains of phenobarbitone and go to bed. After sitting up in bed for half an hour I began to feel better, and eventually went off into a normal sleep. Next morning I felt very limp, but my headache only returned slightly, and had disappeared altogether within a week. I had no further attacks of panic at that time, but felt vaguely anxious, with some palpitation on exertion. After a month I was quite back to normal. I had no investigations apart from sinus X-ray, and no one made any positive suggestion about what had been the matter.

During the next four months I was perfectly well, and, at the age of 44, undertook a strenuous Alpine scrambling holiday. One night in August I woke up with the same feelings of palpitation and panic, which again passed off in half an hour. I had another attack a fortnight later, and thereafter felt anxious during most evenings and could only go to sleep by sitting up in bed and sliding down later. I became afraid of the dark and had to keep a light on. One night in September, whilst on a visit to a relative, I did not sleep until after 7 a.m., in spite of taking seconal, 90 mgm, which only made my anxiety greater. Fortunately, I never had a night as bad as that again.

At the end of September I was left alone for a week-end, while my mother and sister went off to a wedding. I started to cry whilst I was getting myself some supper, and continued for most of the rest of the evening. In desperation I called on a psychiatrist friend, who suggested that I needed a change of environment, without being more specific.

After this I was rather better for two months, although I still had evening anxiety. Then I had one or two days when I had symptoms all day, and I consulted a psychiatrist at a teaching hospital who told me without any hesitation that I had an endogenous depression. He reassured me about the outlook and prescribed sodium amytal, 60 mgm at 3 and 5 p.m. and 180 mgm at 8 p.m. He told me that I could take up to 720 mgm in 24 hours without any worry, if this proved necessary.

For the next seven months I tolerated my symptoms, much helped by the treatment. I did take two 180 mgm capsules within a few hours on one or two days, and an extra 120 mgm at night quite often. A monthly visit to the psychiatrist for reassurance was also helpful.

Following his advice I arranged to carry out another projected Alpine holiday next June. But when the morning came for departure I could not face it and had a prolonged attack of crying. A course of E.C.T. was ordered, and I had two treatments before going away for a fortnight with my mother to visit relatives. I felt very ill during this holiday. I had no interest in anything, and during the next two months, while I was having treatment, I remember rather the few odd periods of an hour or two when I felt relaxed and comfortable, standing out against a background of misery. I managed to continue work, and was much better when actually talking to people and concentrating on them rather than myself.

I completed eight E.C.T. treatments, after which my general mood was much better. I could take an interest in a number of things and my sexual feelings returned. I was still anxious in the evenings and had difficulty with sleeping. Gradually my bad days became fewer, though one or two were as bad as any. I had my last attack of crying in January 1957, and continued taking sodium amytal regularly until February 1958, after an abortive attempt to give it up in the previous autumn. I found, as the psychiatrist had assured me, that I felt no inclination to take the drug once my anxiety had departed.

Since 1958 I have had attacks of anxiety at times, usually not more than twice a year, though I had several in the summer of 1960, associated with temporary giddiness. A precipitating factor has been excessive exertion. I also had persistence of an exaggeration of a previous tendency to claustrophobia, affecting me in any circumstance in which I cannot get out at will, such as in aircraft, trains, and sometimes public occasions. This has subsided gradually over the past six years. I have never again had difficulty in sleeping.

A paternal grandfather and first cousin committed suicide, but the former was senile and the latter had some exogenous cause. There is no family history of mental or nervous disorder otherwise.

Prior to my illness I had always understood that depression and anxiety were two separate conditions, the former likely to be endogenous and the latter due to some environmental or other factor. In accounts of phobic, or, as frequently and unkindly termed "neurotic" depression, it is described as predominantly reactive. In my own case I am convinced that there was some toxic origin. The headache at onset was accompanied by slight pyrexia, and I cannot separate the preliminary brief attack from the later prolonged one. I was interested to read an article in "New Scientist" in 1968, dealing with the metabolism of lactic acid in anxiety states; this seemed to have a bearing on anxiety after unusual exertion.

When considering hypochondriacal states I am sure that the most important distinction is between the motivated and the unmotivated. If the patient gains from his symptoms and the cause for this cannot be removed no treatment is likely to be effective. Where the patient is previously of stable personality, the right treatment is satisfying to everybody.

The approach and general management is the most important. I have learnt that appreciation on the part of the doctor that the symptoms, however "mild" to him, are agonizing to the patient, must be the first point of contact. Next comes firm assurance that a cure is inevitable in time.

In symptomatic treatment, sufficient hypnotic to produce regular sleep is essential. For daytime sedation I have found nothing better than sodium amytal. I tried Meproba, which had little effect, and Drinamyl, which excited me without sedation The patient should be assured that he can safely take a sufficient dose of the drug prescribed, and that no difficulties will be created about repetition of the prescription.

More specifically, I found that E.C.T. benefited my depression of mood and lack of interest, but did not have a great effect on my anxiety. Whilst undergoing it I had frequent olfactory hallucinations, imagining vaguely unpleasant smells in various places where I went. I presume that some effect on the temporal lobes was responsible for this. I never noticed any defect of memory.

I appreciate that today my illness would be treated with a monoamine oxidase inhibitor, and that it would carry a much more favourable prognosis both for duration and severity.

I believe that patients are often wrongly kept off work with depressive illnesses. I found that keeping to a steady routine was helpful, and that concentrating on other peoples' symptoms kept my own more in the background. I was at my worst when on holiday, and very much worse when left alone. Whereas I had previously enjoyed solitude, I needed someone at hand to talk to all the time.

My personal definition which can be understood by every lay person is to call it "Blue Monday" disease, multiplied a hundred times in intensity and length of time. Like rheumatism and gout, the former is one turn of the vice on a joint and the latter three turns of the vice. At its worst depression is a semi-paralysis physical and mental, with varying lengths of time — years, months, weeks.

There are endogenous and exogenous causes. Some psychiatrists think there is no difference in symptoms when you have an intense depression from either cause. That is not my personal experience. I developed a detached retina in 1962 due to my own and other doctors' mistakes, and felt depressed with this disaster, but not as severely as I have had with my own frequent, recurrent attacks of unknown origin. Now exogenous causes are things like some crippling disease or death of a beloved one, or loss of one's job or fortune. This does not apply to me. It didn't apply in my brother's case either. He became a doctor and a successful paediatrician, coming from the same environment. He is 10 years younger than I. My best friend's wife, who is tremendously clever, said that it could never have happened in her family, also poor and originally from Lithuania, because the parents were extremely interested in all things, their business, economics, science and politics and discussed all these varied subjects with the children, four of them. They became outstanding in many careers, medicine, physics, agricultural economics, singing. I have quite a number of hobbies, bridge, bowls, reading — medical and otherwise.

I was born in Lithuania, in a small village, and arrived in South Africa in 1910 at the age of eight years. We lived in a semi-slum area in Cape Town, well-known throughout South Africa and its neighbourhood in Cape Town as District Six. It was mostly occupied at that time by Jewish immigrants from Russia. Two streets, Buitenkant and Maynard, produced an enormous number of outstanding people, professors, two Mayors of Cape Town, a large number of doctors and specialists, lawyers, engineers and extremely successful businessmen.

I became depressed at university, where I spent eight years.
Then I spent a happy year as junior house surgeon at Kimberley,
still not interested in medicine, but enjoying life, women, bridge,
tennis, and became depressed again when I returned to Cape
Town and started practice there. I failed, and then tried another
place, a coloured and poor white area, Parow and Elsie River,
eight miles outside Cape Town. Here at least I made a living, but
not a good one. Anyway, it allowed me to help my parents,
three sisters and brothers at school, and my father struggling in
business. I married, sold my practice in Parow, and left for overseas to specialise in pediatrics, and to take my London M.R.C.P.
The teaching in London was outstanding and wonderful, and
highly specialised. Here I first became intensely interested in
medicine, but I was still depressed and merely thought of myself
as an introvert with an inadequate personality. I failed the
London and then tried the Edinburgh M.R.C.P. and passed it
first time. I then returned to South Africa, and after three
months paediatrics I returned to general practice, in which I
had been partially successful. I was depressed most of the time
and consulted various psychiatrists.

The first psychiatrist was a full-time doctor at the Pretoria
Mental Hospital. He diagnosed depression with elated phases.
He lauded the possession of the latter, saying some of the
greatest geniuses in all branches of human endeavour had this
condition, and that they did their best work only when they
were elated, and that I was fortunate to have this and I must put
up with the depressive stage. He said there was no treatment
except the new shock therapy, with the dangers of death and
fractured vertebrae.

My second psychiatrist was more careful and understanding.
He put my trouble down to the change from school to university,
to my having chosen the wrong profession, and to poor home
environment and possibly to some endogenous causes, some
chemical change in the blood not yet discovered. He warned
me about the elated periods, almost a delusion of grandeur, and
pointed out that I was no genius, judging by my attainments so
far in Pretoria, medical or otherwise, and advised me that I must
restrain myself at all costs, even if I felt in a mood to be the life
and soul of any party. Treatment was to be sedatives only, and
no shock therapy for doctors, as it severely affected the memory
and was only a palliative. My condition, he said, was nearer a
psychosis than a neurosis. In 1950 the attacks became recurrent,
on gradually and off gradually, lasting about three months and
followed by elated periods of about seven days. My first very

short elated period was in 1935, but it returned only from 1940
onwards. He hoped one day they would discover something
that could reverse the duration of my alternating depressions
and elations to three months' elation and three weeks' depression,
which in fact is my condition since 1960.

I went to my third psychiatrist, as my depressions were
continuing and getting me down. I had three months of utter
misery and then a short break of three weeks. He immediately
advised shock therapy. The first time I had one only but did
not continue because of fear. The second time I had six treatments over a period of two weeks. I felt better after this, but
the depression returned in a month's time. The third time I
spent two weeks in the clinic and had six shocks with no
improvement. That was the last shock therapy I ever had. It
caused a shocking memory defect for six weeks. I could not
remember the name of the simplest drug, or disease, or people's
names.

My fourth psychiatrist was a new neighbour in my medical
centre. He was very kind and helpful and we became very friendly.
This was the phase of the new drugs, M.A.O. and later the tri-
cyclic drugs. We experimented with all. I told him I was prepared
to be a guinea pig. This was 1956-58. They were a tremendous
improvement on any previous treatment. I tried everything,
even to having my outstanding ears corrected by a plastic surgeon.
This certainly diminished by depression by about 10%. Then I
tried contact lenses to replace my thick glasses. This was
disastrous, as it led to a detached retina. My psychiatrist approved
thoroughly of anything that improved one's appearance.

When this psychiatrist moved to another building, my fifth
psychiatrist was a younger man. I found him the best of all. He
seemed to understand the whole condition as if he had it himself, which he told me later he had, but in a less severe form than
mine. I still use him.

Psychiatrist six: I asked advice from a young American
professor of psychiatry at one of our annual medical congresses
in Durban in 1959. He lectured on the new psychotropic drugs.
He advised only shock therapy. He was rather abrupt, saying he
had come to South Africa to lecture, not to attend private
patients.

Psychiatrist seven: a similar experience befell me when I inter-
viewed another professor of psychiatry also on a lecture tour to
South Africa. He also was abrupt at first but later softened. He
said he did first an endocrinological survey in his hospital clinic.
I had myself tested here, but the result was negative.

Psychiatrist eight: a London psychiatrist, when I was very deeply depressed at the Moorfields Eye Hospital, London. This was my deepest depression, and lasted four weeks owing to both endogenous and exogenous causes. He prescribed Nardil and Librium and I recovered in three days to hypomanic heights. He was the only doctor who charged me in London — £36 for three to four consultations. The bill stated that this was a 20% reduction as I was a medical colleague. He said all recurrences would be successfully treated in the same way. He made no suggestion for prevention of attacks.

Psychiatrist nine: I wrote to a famous London psychiatrist but he could not give advice as he was too far away.

Psychiatrist ten: I was deeply retarded. My brother and sister were relieved when I left them after a week, and moved to an hotel. This psychiatrist gave me Parnate tablets. He took no adequate history and did not suggest seeing me again. He also gave me lithium tablets. Both failed hopelessly.

There has been a continuous improvement in the years 1960-1970. My depression now averages two to four weeks and my elated normal phases six to twelve weeks. At the moment I take one tablet of Anafranal and one to two tablets of Valium, 2 to 5 mg. I started with tablets of amytriptyline (25 mg) three times a day for a few days, then changed to intramuscular injection of amytriptyline, 2 ml, for seven to fourteen days. When not better I take Anafranal, first one then two at night, then add Valium, 5 mg, three times a day, and this brakes my last depression. I have three weeks of the usual utter misery, of being a moron, semi-paralysed and retarded. I have some side effects from the amytriptyline and other drugs. My mouth and nose become very dry and crusted, I become constipated, and my vision less clear, but at least I am out of misery. I wake very early, 2.30 to 5 a.m., when I do my best reading or writing, medically or otherwise.

My wife says she has had an awful life with me, and I heartily agree with her. I don't know whether I would have tolerated her if she had such an illness. She is a well-educated woman, and is and always has been a great reader. She is an extrovert and was secretary and then Chairman of the local Christmas Stamp Fund for many years. She gets on very well with all races and the best people, and has become a successful travel agent in recent years, when the children grew up, going overseas every year, and she has been everywhere except South America and the communist countries. We have two sons, tall, good-looking and both successful extroverts.

I wanted to form Depression Clubs with local, national and international branches of the Mental Health Society, on the lines of the World Diabetic, Coronary and Peptic Ulcer Clubs. I tried to interest a few people in such a project, but it is not a popular name and subject. It is too close to insanity. Perhaps if we called it the "Blue Monday Club" it may have more appeal and not frighten people away. One hides such a disease and does not advertise it, says my wife. I disagree entirely. If you call it by a more euphemistic term life will be easier for the well and sick partners, because you will have an adequate and not morbid explanation for erratic behaviour and cancellation of appointments. One cannot make definite appointments, be on committees, take part in debates, or speak at social functions, as one never knows when the depression will come on and lay one low for several weeks. One could then form friendships too, as others will appreciate your recurrent ill-health. People tolerate the recurrent ill-health due to peptic ulcers, diabetes, hypertension, but not near-mental disease.

There should be no such thing as separate mental hospitals, except for the permanent, hopeless psychotics. It should form a division of a general hospital, like any other division, and should have an annex for occupational therapy.

I say there is no alcoholism, only depression. My psychiatric colleagues dispute this. They say that in alcoholism there is 10% depression, 90% inadequate personality. I cannot accept this contention. Some of the finest people, great sportsmen, professors and lecturers at university, members of every profession, successful tradesmen and business executives, become alcoholics. Are they all inadequate personalities? If the strain is great enough, any personality will fail and become depressed and look for relief. It is such an utterly devastating, demoralising disease that you either commit suicide or look for relief in drink or drugs. I have quite a number of successes in treating alcoholics as depressives. I can treat them by myself if they live near me or visit my office twice daily. I give them two to three intramuscular injections of 2 ml amytriptyline (also oral Limbritol) for 7-14 days, then once daily for 7 days, then on alternate days for a week, then twice weekly. They have to be watched and treated for about six weeks. They become happy and lose all interest in alcohol, even if they surreptitiously continue on the drink for the first few weeks. Like sufferers from any other chronic recurrent disease, they must be treated for life. I asked a psychiatrist running an alcoholic clinic to let me try out my experiment for several weeks, but I have heard nothing more from him. Even the worst and most confirmed alcoholic feels better when he is told it is not a sinful disease, nor immoral nor due to an inadequate personality, but to depression, which has caused him to look for relief from his misery. A few patients have stopped drinking without treatment, after hearing this explanation. We will never solve the alcoholism problem by our present methods, but treat it as a depression and I see great success, as there are better and improved drugs all the time. It is still utter hell while the depression lasts. I try to break my depression in two days, naturally allowing for one or two weeks from the gradual descent from normality to depression, with the latest treatment by dibenzepin drip. You go into a nursing home at 7 p.m., have the drip for twelve hours, and leave the next morning at 7 a.m. You must be watched by a nurse all the time, your blood pressure and pulse measured and the needle prevented from slipping.

# Chapter XIV

# Disseminated Sclerosis

If a sufferer from this unhappy complaint were comparing his symptoms with those of a medical textbook he must not expect them to tally. Some items in the book would almost certainly be missing from his laundry list.

The first of my own symptoms seemed innocent enough and I regarded it more in the light of a normal physiological response. As a medical officer in a tropical region during the War, it was a custom each morning whenever possible to congregate and partake of immoderate quantities of tea. Within half an hour of these occasions I developed urgency of micturition. Convincing myself that the excesses were dictated by social rather than needful requirements, a "cure" was simply and rapidly effected by considerably reducing my intake.

Three or four months earlier I had been unfortunate enough on leaving the hospital in the darkness after a spell of duty, to fall from a steep flight of steps in the grounds. Instead of my feet coming in contact with soft earth, my loin struck a low concrete wall with full force and I was promptly returned, a shocked stretcher casualty, to take a patient's view of all that went on inside. I was quite content to settle for three fractured transverse processes and after a few weeks stepped briskly from the portals. All seemed well again.

Soon, however, owing to serious family illness, I was anxious to return to the U.K. and was given the opportunity of a passage home.

The urgency of micturition now seemed of little consequence and in fact had been brought under control. The thought of reporting the matter, when more was at stake, never crossed my mind and the symptom was completely forgotten. Little did I realise that years later this was to cost me a possible disablement pension. The creed of the watch-dogs of our public expenditure is "No confirmatory evidence, no pension". It is comforting to know we have such devoted guards and I only wish their numbers were greater in other Government Departments.

I well remember one spring morning whilst brushing my teeth in the bathroom, gazing into the mirror over the basin to see if my face looked as odd as it felt. A sharply delineated numbness and tingling had suddenly developed in the right half of my head. My immediate thought was of a Bell's palsy and I felt relieved when I saw a perfectly symmetrical face looking back at me.

Well at least, the mischief hadn't started yet. But it couldn't be anything of importance; I felt so fit. The list that morning was long and tedious and there was no time to give the matter further consideration. On returning in the evening my face felt perfectly normal and has remained so ever since.

I sincerely hope the cases of "trigeminal sensory neuropathy" recently described in one of the medical journals will not turn out as mine did.

That summer as I was gardening I tripped over a concatenation of roots stretched across a path and sprained my right ankle. The pain slowly subsided and I gradually ceased to hobble around. Some months later whilst taking a brisk uphill walk to collect the car from a garage, the toe-cap of my right shoe kept grazing the pavement. Confound that foot! It hasn't recovered completely yet, I thought. I'd better see an orthopod, he might advise me about those painful callosities on my feet at the same time.

Mr. Calcaneum, whom I consulted, was a benevolent old gentleman who considered his speciality sufficient unto itself and sorely resented the intrusion of any extraneous medical condition. For a down to earth fracture, arthritis or bunion he was without equal.

The consultation concluded with a thorough inspection of my footwear and a pair of ingenious inner-soles was prescribed. I found these a boon but the metatarsal bar something of a hindrance. So too, was the pair of shoes with the soles raised on their outer sides; it was like performing a music-hall act just to step out in them. However, by avoiding steep inclines and wearing the magic inner-soles normal locomotion was re-established.

The summer months of the following year were unusually fine and sunny and few places could have looked more attractive than Harrogate. The B.M.A. had happily chosen this salubrious spot for their Annual Meeting.

I was anxious to attend the section dealing with my particular subject, whether to learn, to contribute or just for the pleasure of the occasion I cannot recall; probably all three. It involved a long car journey to accomplish this in the one day I had set aside for the purpose and I was away to an early start. The sun's glare was almost hurtful to my eyes throughout the drive and, worse still, I had left my sun-glasses behind. On the homeward run, with many miles still to cover in a steadily fading light, I developed diplopia and had to complete the journey at snail-pace with one hand occluding an eye. It was an experience I shall long remember and lost no time in consulting the experienced ophthalmologist at our hospital. I mentioned nothing of the incidents which had already occurred as I thought them trivial and unconnected.

The lenses he prescribed contained a pyramid and overcame the optical imbalance satisfactorily but the orthoptic exercises ordered were time consuming and of little benefit. There was never pallor of the temporal half of the discs and the fine horizontal nystagmus had, I think, been present as long as I can remember.

I was now happily set up again and went about my business with a new zeal but, two years later, on a rain-free afternoon we took a cliff walk which was to prove my undoing. During the latter half of the expedition my daughter, a toddler at the time, tired and had to be carried. With her legs over my shoulders we traversed the rough ground but after a time my own legs became so unsteady that it was dangerous to continue. She completed the journey on my son's shoulders while I stumbled disconsolately back to the hotel.

For some time before, my sphincters had not been as dependable as good sphincters ought to be, and I began to piece the jigsaw together. Unequal, exaggerated knee-jerks tended to confirm my worst suspicions and I spent the rest of the evening with unhappy thoughts.

On returning home I consulted a neurologist and full-scale investigation in hospital revealed the truth. To comfort me the kindly old gentleman told of many who had survived to pensionable age. Sentence having been duly passed, the remainder of my stay in hospital became a whirl of therapy, hypnotic tablets and confused actuarial calculations. Under these conditions little in the way of serious planning could be worked out and I was glad to get home.

There was still much to be done and I could see a great deal would depend on financial considerations. The children's education and the melancholy thought of premature retirement pointed to the importance of earning whatever I could for as long as possible.

Fortunately there were no further dramatic developments — just a gradual deterioration of locomotion and balance.

My work was largely concerned with sitting on a stool and turning knobs in the correct sequence and at the right time.

Visits to the wards or walking the length of the table to set up a pedal drip became embarrassing towards the end. I learned that by anticipating difficulties crises rarely occurred. Fortunately, the gods dealt leniently with me and I was able to carry on in this way for a further ten years.

In view of the protean manifestations of this disease I feel, as an observer from within, that the standard medical textbooks make a remarkably good job of the diagnosis.

Though no specific treatment at present exists, adequate management can make life more worthwhile.

For the chairbound a functional home is the very heart of successful management. It must be on one floor and preferably have a view. A bleak future can thus be quite transformed.

The gloom inherent in the mind of the physically incapacitated can in large measure be dissipated before it rubs off with demoralising effect on the family.

This tailor-made bungalow is set in the side of a valley, and beyond the river there is a wide mountainous panorama. I always feel it is a better place than we would have normally retired to, but, of course, that may only be a piece of self-deception.

There is not the tendency in the country to keep up with the Joneses — an important consideration for those in retirement. (A narrow escape for us as it happens, for in this part, of all surnames, Jones is by far the most numerous.)

Steps have been entirely eliminated from the bungalow and slightly wider doors permit uninterrupted passage of the chair without grazing the knuckles. Under-floor heating has proved a great boon on cold days for I must now regard my feet as circulatorily under privileged.

Three items are vital in the bathroom. A lavatory according enthronement and abdication with dignity, a waist-high tubular metal wall-rail close to the washbasin and a shower-tray below floor level containing that sine qua non, the Remploy chair-bath. This should be connected to a thermally controlled water supply. Another wall-bar above the tray facilitates transfer from chair to chair. These aids can be installed in quite a small space leaving adequate room for both conventional bath and wheel-chair manoeuvres. Moreover, they make for complete independence.

Bowel and bladder disciplines can prevent disasters, both domestic and medical. A satisfactory state of colonic automation can be brought about by taking a bulk laxative such as All-Bran.

An incompletely emptied bladder if allowed to pass unnoticed can lead to a serious condition and attention to this point is

Well worth while. Micturition in a standing position before retiring pays good dividends. Holding the wall-bar in the bathroom with one hand and a plastic receptacle with the other is not such a remarkable acrobatic feat as it sounds. I complete all drinking for the day by 6.0 p.m. (with certain reservations). The pangs of a distended bladder in the paling dawn are at all costs to be avoided.

The soothing effect of an electric blanket and a firm but gentle mattress should not be underestimated though the prospect of going to bed — like the policeman's lot — is not a happy one. Heavy blankets drawn tightly over grossly weakened lower limbs are unendurable and should be replaced by loosely applied cellular-woollen ones. If unperturbed by falling out of bed in the dead of night, a single divan is all right though my own preference is for a double one.

Soon after finding a relaxed position my legs begin to ache or the part of my heel pressing on the under sheet becomes unbearably painful.

This calls for a tedious reshuffle but a similar state builds up after a few minutes and the merry-go-round continues.

About midnight the Battle of Adductor Predominance commences and with clarion-calls of cramp and violent reflex action, the lower limbs are in a state of turmoil throughout the night. These distressing interludes can be alleviated to a certain extent by taking a sedative — and indeed after a succession of disturbed nights one is driven to this course — but in the limitless situation posed by D.S., where the slippery slopes of drug dependence may soon be reached, a critical judgement has to be made between the lesser of two evils.

That much-needed drug — a neuromuscular blocking agent in tablet form — has still to be discovered though there are many misrepresentations put on the market by lesser known drug firms.

Unless pedicure is regularly carried out an unfortunate laceration could well be inflicted on the feet during a violent spasm.

"Do it yourself physiotherapy" earns an important place, I feel, in the home management of D.S. Passive abduction of the legs and tiptoe exercises can be practised at the bathroom wall-rail as a batsman practises his strokes at the nets. Holding the rail with the hands and prising oneself up from the chair the legs are then extended. On a firm smooth floor, with shoes side by side, the feet are gradually shuffled apart so that the legs form an isosceles. A 24″ base is good, an equilateral formation even better — particularly if the position can be held for five minutes.

I haven't ventured beyond that distance for fear of doing myself a mischief!

Adiposity must be a great trial in this condition and militates against successful management. Therein lies the importance of watching the calories. Everything possible should be done to minimise the amount of heaving the arms are called upon to do. Personally I endeavour not to exceed 1200 cals. per day — apart, of course, from high days and holidays when the diet is conveniently forgotten. Even so, by evening arthralgic pain is making its appearance in my shoulders. This, I find, is effectively controlled by Prednisolone, 5 mg nocte. The drug is so valuable in this context that I have taken it for almost ten years without alteration of dosage or ill-effect.

One of the unfortunate effects of this complaint is the increased proneness to accident.

At the beginning of my retirement I was altogether too venturesome and had a number of falls but only one, fortunately, of any consequence.

I then injured my shoulder and it was two years before I was able to use it fully again without pain. For the greater part of that time my incapacity was virtually trebled and I began to realise the importance of maintaining in good working order what powers are left. I was never a candidate for belt and braces but now feel that risks are quite unjustifiable.

More lavishly cushioned buttocks than my own are in the habit of suffering discomfort from prolonged immobility in the sitting position so I make no apology for the square of Dunlopillo secreted between this part of my anatomy and the canvas seat of the wheel-chair. For good measure I also transfer in the evening to the luxury of a deeply upholstered "High-seat" chair which involves the use of a walking-aid. The type I use — the Fordham's variety — has a folding frame and is supported on three wheels, the front one possessing a cable-brake which can be operated by rotating the right handle-bar grip. This appliance bears much the same resemblance to the old tripod as a greyhound to a hippopotamus.

It might well be assumed that personal whims and preferences occupy the whole of my day; that life is confined to a therapeutic treadmill, the door of which is locked from without, but this would be far from correct. The daily routine once begun coasts along automatically and time is given to less mundane assignments. Correspondence, music, various literary pursuits and gazing out over the valley at the miraculous way in which Nature manages her affairs, all make up a busy day.

increasing intracranial pressure by the Valsalva manoeuvre, to the positioning of the head on the neck, and the grading of pain grades of severity from 0 to 4, particularly asking whether the pain disappears completely to zero between pulsations, affords valuable evidence in the diagnosis of the nature and mechanism of the headache. The answers to these simple questions appear to offer information of considerable value at least in distinguishing between low pressure headache, migraine headache, meningeal headache, cervical origin headache, and head pains due to direct involvement of sensory nerves such as the fifth nerve. To many patients these would be just headaches. To some undiscerning doctors they might be "just a recurrence of the original headache". To me, the comfort given by analysing and understanding the mechanisms of the various head pains was considerable. I at least knew that those pains which appeared after the fifth cranial nerve neuritis and the "meningeal" headache were not due to a relapse of the original pathological state, whatever that was.

I have purposely refrained from describing the features of my illness that were not related to its painful episodes. Nor have I discussed the diagnosis of the cause. Was it encephalitis, was it the "vertebral artery" syndrome or other vascular anomaly, or what else was it?

Subjects more courageous than myself, should they suffer the same type of illness as I suffered, may subject themselves to more lumbar punctures, to intravenous instillation of hypertonic and hypotonic saline, to suspension by the feet, and to other mechanical manoeuvres. My object in describing these head pains to you is to stimulate someone to study in a more thorough way than I did the head pains that may occur during the course of an illness such as mine and in other conditions as well.

## Chapter XXIII

# Infective Hepatitis

Several of us "expatriates" working at a Middle East hospital in the 1950's before the days of routine gamma globulin prophylaxis contracted infective hepatitis sooner or later.

Typically the first few days of my own attack were a mystery — I felt vague malaise, then became feverish with vomiting, lastly bile appeared in the urine and the mystery was over. (One missionary colleague: "I thought I had lost my faith until I turned yellow"!)

The first two weeks of being yellow were not too uncomfortable with no depression, and time for reading at leisure in a single room in a private hospital. Then things went wrong. I could not eat without horrible discomfort afterwards. Thinking that I knew about the liver, I was eating as much protein as I could manage, which was not much, but even non-fatty items like chicken started to cause vile colic and flatus. Now we know that the virus infects the intestine as well as the liver. I might have known. Colic after any food became so severe that I sometimes got out of bed and rolled on the floor. A good nurse provided warm peppermint water which helped a bit. Eating nearly nothing helped more; a little toast and jam, and fruit such as those marvellous water-melons.

My kind physician gave me intravenous glucose — an ampoule daily, during this phase, and I also had intramuscular vitamin B. I expect they helped. A consultant advised tetracycline to alter the intestinal flora, which seemed to stop the colic, but the effect did not last. He also noted ecchymoses on my shins which cleared after a dose of vitamin K. One cause of pain was constipation. The relief of an enema has to be experienced to be believed. I had several.

Three or four weeks from onset I was a deep orange colour and could smell bile in my breath all the time. There was a "whirring" sensation in my liver which intensified in the afternoon indicating that the disease was more active then. As the swollen liver cells caused intra-hepatic obstruction each evening the surge of bile in the circulation brought an overwhelming

feeling of black depression — the melancholia of the ancients.
Then each night the itching of this obstructive phase became
maddening.

How welcome was that draught of chloral at 10 p.m.
giving two or three hours of oblivion before the wakeful hours
to dawn. The virus activity seems to subside in those small hours
which provided an opportunity to eat a bit. Later an ex-R.A.F.
officer told me how he and his comrades used to raid their ward
kitchen at night in India. Being hungry in the small hours does
not suit a rigid ward routine so I used to hoard food in my locker
and have a 4 a.m. meal, although one delightful night-sister discovered my need and produced welcome succour. Breakfast, likewise, could be managed better than other meals. Lunch was too
late and I had to refuse tempting items from then on, for otherwise I incurred the penalty of later discomfort and colic and
reduced sleep. Sleeplessness left me exhausted and did me no
good, but eventually I learnt to alternate days of eating a bit,
which I felt I needed, and days of eating almost nothing, which
gave me more rest.

One difficulty about sleep is that I normally sleep lying prone.
With a high concentration of bile in one's circulation the effect
of it on one's brain is intensified when one lies flat. The resulting
increase of depression made sleep impossible. It is more comfortable propped up with a backrest, as the nurses knew, but if
this is not one's usual sleeping position one does need a sedative.
Chloral tastes horrible but followed by a boiled sweet and then a
tooth-brushing it did the trick. Other sedatives were contra-
indicated because of the liver dysfunction.

One lesson I learnt — to drink enough fluids. Sweet drinks
were sickly so I squeezed limes into water and added glucose.
This was delicious and saved my life. I drank jugs of it and
gallons of water. I could reduce my worst symptoms — the wave
of depression and the itching — by washing bile out of my circulation by a really large fluid intake. A whole jugful of water
drunk straight from the jug at night reduced the itching enough
to let me sleep fitfully. A full bladder was more easily relieved
than itching limbs. Methyl testosterone tablets did not seem to
help the pruritus nor did an anti-histamine. I steeled myself not
to scratch but one night I dreamt that I was a cock and dug my
claws into my shins until they bled! This aggravated the itching
for quite a while.

It is difficult to understand the depression unless one has
experienced it. A nice G.P. who had a severe attack of jaundice
himself put his head round the door one day and said as much

which gave me enormous comfort. But my mental symptoms did not stop at depression. I was garrulous at times, pouring out nonsense to bewildered visitors, and when alone my mind raced continuously. In a single room I felt desperately lonely but fellow patients in an open ward would have found me a difficult companion. I think the mental symptoms were aggravated sometimes by hypoglycaemia: I remember feeling suddenly better after a glucose drink.

When very ill I longed for visitors but could not keep up a conversation for many minutes. It was best for me if they came and just sat for a while, but naturally this did not often happen. Visitors like to talk, and this could be tiring. For a time I was forbidden all visitors except for my wife and this was obviously right at that stage. Rest is all-important for infective hepatitis. It took me time to realise, for instance, that getting up to have a bath was not a good idea. Like many people I dislike "doing nothing" and kept wanting to read, write letters, practice typing and so on. Later I sat out in a chair in my room each afternoon but for weeks that was all that I could manage without undue fatigue. However once I learnt to relax both physically and mentally I began to improve more rapidly. This was not easily learnt. A colleague who asked what was my idea of the treatment for infective hepatitis was told "prayer and fasting". (The fasting, of course, should not be more than necessity decrees.)

Finally, nearly three months from onset, with the jaundice fading, I was promised transfer to England once my serum bilirubin was normal. I made sure that it was normal by taking a large drink of water before the blood was taken. In hospital in London a few days later I put on two pounds per day on a high protein, moderate carbohydrate and low fat diet — notably great slices of lean meat for breakfast. Iron corrected a slight anaemia. My liver function tests were normal, so after two weeks I was discharged to my family in the countryside, feeling jubilant, but wobbly. It was another six weeks or so before I could manage to walk much, then I began to feel my normal strength returning and was fit enough six months from onset to travel back. We were just in time for the Suez crisis.

I had another eight years working in tropical Africa after that with only two or three days of minor illness. Fortunately the liver has powers of regeneration.

The first two weeks of February 1970 I spent in Austria on a skiing holiday. It was my second such holiday and I had found it invigorating after a long period of general surgery. I returned home to take up combined clinical and academic work but by the fifth day I started to feel listless with complete aversion from food. I struggled on feeling that it may be just a "back to work" or "change of job" reaction. After 3 days I began to be troubled with a generalised urticarial skin rash. This was most marked on the upper anterior trunk, with fleeting erythematous blotches surrounding very itchy weals. I now began to experience upper abdominal discomfort accompanied by fullness and marked borborygmi. The rash disappeared in 48 hours and by this time listlessness, lethargy, anorexia and insomnia were extreme. For the first time, now five days since my first symptoms, I noticed darkening of the urine. I had some biochemical checks the following morning which showed a serum bilirubin of 4 mg with enzyme (SGOT and SGPT) estimations over 800 units. After a sleepless night with nausea and vomiting I agreed to go into hospital for about 10 days, by which time I thought the extreme sickness would be over and I would be on the way to recovery. It did in fact turn out instead to be 10 weeks.

For the first 2-3 weeks I did not care what happened or whether I got better or not. I had such constant nausea and pain, felt not only in the epigastrium and right hypochondrium but radiating to the inter-scapular region of the back and both shoulders. It was so severe at times that I felt convinced I must have gall stones in spite of the history and biochemistry pointing to an "infective" illness. Aversion from food was peculiar. I was not hungry and yet at times I would desire some delicacy, which on being produced would be pushed aside like the regular meals. I lost over 2 stones in weight in these early weeks and bilirubin levels climbed to over 20 mg. I detected recurring crops of xanthomata starting a few days after admission to hospital. At first bright yellow they faded to a dark brown, then to a dull green and finally disappeared by desquamation. They were pin-head in size and localised to the fingers of both hands — most marked on the index and middle fingers where they occurred in rows on the sides of the digit distal to the proximal inter-phalangeal joints. Constipation was extreme during this period.

About the third week of my illness I started to feel a little better and took some interest in my surroundings. I could tolerate fluids well and also a little food. The serum enzymes had started to fall rapidly but the bilirubin level fell but little. I now entered a cholestatic phase when the greatest trial was an unremitting pruritus. Although generalised, the palms of the hands, the soles of the feet and the interdigital clefts were the

main focus of attention throughout the long hours of the night.
I found the perpendicular rails on the foot of the hospital bed
an excellent weapon with which to scratch the plantar interdigital clefts. A little help was obtained from phenobarbitone
1 grain at night, sodium bicarbonate baths twice daily and
cholestyramine twice daily. The Questran brand of the latter I
found very constipating but much more palatable than an
earlier preparation.

This cholestatic phase lasted about 6 weeks and was certainly
the most trying period of my illness. Many enquiries were made
by my attending physicians about the possibility of drugs causing
my hepatitis, but this cause was completely ruled out. Steroid
therapy was recommended by some as a diagnostic "wash-out"
and by others as a "therapeutic" measure. In preparation for a
course a preliminary barium study was made of the upper gastro-
intestinal tract. The procedure did not upset me at all, but
getting rid of the barium from both the bowel and the subsequent water toilet was quite a feat. Then, to everybody's amazement, a further biochemical check showed a fall in the bilirubin
level. I was spared treatment and this biochemical improvement
continued slowly but steadily till normal figures were reached
about 4 months after the onset of illness.

The accompanying mental lethargy of hepatitis is a very
definite feature. At first I was too sick to be able to read, too
sick to concentrate and too sick even to care. About the fourth
week a hearty colleague gave me a good laugh and this I regard
as my first step out of mental apathy. Thereafter I took some
interest in reading but concentration was very limited. I found
jig-saw puzzles good occupational therapy at this stage. In later
months I played scrabble with my nephew and nieces. At first I
could scarcely formulate any words but a steadily increasing
score (used as an index of mental concentration) was a great
encouragement to me.

It is now 7 months since I took ill. I returned to work at the
end of August, putting in about 4 hours of non-clinical work
each day. I find that even this is mentally and physically exhausting. I still require about 14 hours bed rest every 24 hours. My
weight has returned almost to normal and my appetite is quite
good. One persisting complaint is an episodic urticarial rash of
arms and legs which I treat symptomatically with systemic
Piriton and topical hydrocortisone cream. A pigmented
"waterline" across my forehead about 1 inch from a receding
hair line is now the only evident brand mark of my past
illness.

On looking back I can say that throughout it all the greatest
distractions to me personally as a patient were the dermatologi-
cal manifestations of the disease.

Skin Rash
        XANTHOMATA
                PRURITUS
                        Urticarial Skin Rash
                                Pigmented Water-line

| 0 | 1 | 2 | 3 | 4 | 5 | 6 | 7 |
|---|---|---|---|---|---|---|---|

Duration in Months

Certainly the experiences of life teach the most unforgettable
lessons.

In the autumn of 1946, then a male aged forty, I developed
catarrhal jaundice with an abrupt onset. One day the urine was
brownish, the stool clay-coloured, and there was deep jaundice
of the skin.

There was no obvious source of infection. Although many of
the military establishments in the neighbourhood that invited
me regularly to entertainments and that supplied quite a number
of patients to my E.M.S. hospital had been closed, a few, such
as prisoner-of-war camps, lingered, but I cannot remember
whether I was visiting near enough to the onset for any
connection to be assumed. It had been found in similar cases
from these units that the causative organisms had a life cycle
usually of forty-two days, but sometimes only twenty-one and
rarely just ten days.

Being then superintendent and surgeon of the then County
General Hospital, Worksop, it was clearly needful forthwith to
be seen by one of the consulting physicians about my duties.
He said there was no need to go to bed, that I could continue
my administrative work (which involved less than half normal
working hours and entailed little else than office work), but
that all clinical work (normally ward rounds and operating
sessions) should be suspended. The County Council accepted his
recommendations, and allowed me to use its petrol coupons for
motoring the two miles between my home and the hospital.

As would be expected, the only symptom resulted from the
hepatic dysfunction and consisted of flatulent indigestion. There
was vague abdominal discomfort, with considerable bowel movement, much wind, and rather loose motions.

In a few days it became obvious that lunches, teas, and suppers exacerbated the indigestion very uncomfortably, but this did not happen after breakfast. A little thought led to the assumption that while enough bile was available in the morning for assisting the proper digestion of breakfasts, there was not time enough for sufficient to be excreted during the few hours between breakfast and subsequent meals. So comparative comfort was achieved by eating substantial breakfasts each day, and thereafter taking plenty of fluid but only a minimal amount of solid food.

At night, however, the abdominal discomfort definitely hindered sleep until again a little thought yielded the idea of converting abdominal breathing to thoracic breathing, thus avoiding the diaphragm pumping the inflamed liver up and down. It was found surprisingly easy to adopt the habit of thoracic breathing, traditionally that of the opposite sex; hepatic excursion was considerably lessened, and thereafter sleep was satisfactory. Also, it should have been predictable that any long period of motoring would involve a fair amount of jolting of the liver, and bring discomfort.

So, after the first week or so, I had learnt to live with the condition with only minor discomfort. Thereafter, my substantial amount of free time was spent mostly in gardening, the weather being fine, and in similar domestic chores.

On the forty-second day from its onset the condition cleared as abruptly as it had begun: the urine that day was clear yellow, the stool brown again, and the jaundice disappeared.

No medicines were recommended or taken. There have been no recurrences and no sequelae. Indeed, with some amusement I noted a life insurance doctor searching my body for a full three-quarters of an hour twenty years later when I was aged sixty, but the result was a first-class life grading.

There was an epidemic in Bahrain at the time. I was Government Surgeon and went to most of the parties that were going. A few weeks before I became ill the navy had a big party for a visiting ship and I was there. Soon after sailing, we heard that 16 of the visiting crew had developed hepatitis. From the timing it seems that they did *not* acquire the infection in Bahrain, but were infectious while on land. Droplet infection when talking or

laughing seems very probable. Sanitation was reasonably good:-
my house was very fly-free but, of course, faecal contamination
is always possible.

For about 3 days I became more and more nauseated. I
vomited most of my meals in spite of taking all the usual simple
remedies mist. As the temperature was $100° - 120°$ in the shade
this was rather disturbing. My consulting room was not air-
conditioned and members of the staff became worried about the
dangers of dehydration. Eventually the anaesthetist arrived with
a saline bottle and transfusion set to give me some fluid before I
left for hospital, but on that day, for the first time I was
jaundiced and my urine contained bile. I was admitted to
hospital.

I had no fever throughout and my liver was never tender or
palpable. I had one pint of saline and then the drip was taken
down.

I was in an air-conditioned room but was allowed to get up
or stay in bed as I liked. I took two showers a day and sat out
in a chair reading or sewing for about half the day.

My chief trouble was extreme and agonising oesophagitis and
gastritis. I was both hungry and thirsty but as soon as I took
anything, even water, I had the most distressing substernal pain.
For the first few days I vomited a good deal and so had hell
while it went down and again as it came back. At no time was I
repelled by food — I wanted it but was really frightened of the
inevitable pain. I felt weak and vaguely ill but had none of the
depression usually described.

My serum bilirubin was estimated daily. The physician wanted
to give me cortisone but I refused as I am very chary of messing
about with hormones. However, when my bilirubin reached
27 mg% I relented and had 200 mg cortisone per day for about
3 days, then 100 for 3 days, then 50 for 2 days then stopped.

I had then been in hospital for exactly 3 weeks, my jaundice
was fading rapidly and I was well enough to go home. On the
day I left hospital I woke to find myself enormously oedematous.
I could hardly open my eyes or mouth, and I looked like a
Michelin tyre advertisement. The physician still sent me home
and I took no medicine at all, but the same night I had a massive
diuresis and excreted a measured 4 lbs weight between going to
bed and taking breakfast next day. My oedema had almost vanished.

I had lost 13 lbs in weight during the illness and was then
eating everything I could get. The oesophagitis faded with the
jaundice. I had three helpings of everything, which was deemed
unfair. My weight returned to 10 stone 2 lbs where it has stayed.

In 2 more weeks, five weeks from the onset, I was back at
full work in hospital.

My liver function tests rapidly returned to normal where
they have stayed ever since. I have never had any trace of a
recurrence, indeed have had no illness of any sort. At 61 I can
still go on to the tennis court after a day in the theatre and
play four sets of singles so my constitution has not notably
suffered.

There are few points of interest in this account, I fear. The
most unpleasant aspect was the vomiting followed by really
severe pain. I had no pruritus, anorexia or constipation (up to
6 bulky stools a day throughout). The 24 hours of oedema was
odd. Was it due to the cortisone or to liver malfunction? In
spite of a pretty high serum bilirubin, there have been no
sequels whatever.


The following is a brief account of an unusually prolonged attack
of infective hepatitis. The onset was very sudden. I went to bed
on the evening of May 17th, 1955, feeling quite normal and
woke up in the early hours of May 18th with the knowledge
that I was running a temperature and feeling as one always does
in such circumstances. My temperature was 101. Before this
sudden onset I had had no warning of what was coming, although,
being wise after the event, there were two prior occurrences, one
of which was possibly only a coincidence, but the second
probably not.

The first incident occurred on April 21st. The previous evening
I had attended a dinner at the Dorchester Hotel and had both
eaten and drunk the normal sort of quantity that is usual on
such occasions. My consumption of wine was strictly moderate
and in no way excessive by any standards. Notwithstanding this,
I woke up next morning with a surprising hangover and feeling
what is colloquially termed "livery". This sensation did not last
long and after I had had some breakfast I felt quite normal.
Although this incident occurred exactly four weeks before the
acute phase started, I understand that the incubation period of
the hepatitis virus is believed to be a long one and the incident
might therefore be significant.

There were no other symptoms until May 16th when I was
completely "off my feed" at lunchtime and found all food distasteful. This sensation also passed off quickly and I was able to
eat a normal meal in the evening. It so happened that that night

I went to the Caledonian Ball which is a very long and strenuous affair lasting from 9 p.m. until 3 a.m. There was a sit-down supper in the middle of the proceedings which I negotiated quite normally, and I survived an unusually strenuous night with no greater degree of tiredness than I would have expected even in normal circumstances. I had no hangover and the following day, May 17th, did a normal day's work and ate meals normally. That night the acute phase started.

There were only two other minor symptoms. One was that on the 16th I had experienced slight earache. This took the form of slight stabs of pain which were only momentary and did not really worry me at all. It may well have been pure coincidence. The second was that I experienced a slight tingling and burning sensation in the skin, particularly on the forearms. This sensation was similar to a very mild degree of sunburn.

The first few days of the acute phase followed the normal pattern of any febrile illness and in the absence of any more positive symptoms, was thought to be 'flu. For the first three days the morning temperature was about 101 and the evening temperature was 102. Although there was as yet no pigmentation of the eyes or skin, pigmentation of the urine was first noticed on May 21st and jaundice was diagnosed. That morning vomiting occurred and again the following morning, but in spite of the weeks of nausea that were to follow these were the only two occasions on which vomiting actually occurred. During this high temperature period I was in a dopey condition and was virtually unable to eat solid food. It was a great effort to drink an adequate quantity of glucose in solution. For the next three or four days pigmentation of the skin and eyes became marked and the temperature tended to return to normal except in the evening, when it usually went up a little.

In the second week a stage of stability was reached during which I felt less ill and was able to eat a little solid food. In view of this and having been told that the normal course of the disease lasted a matter of three or four weeks, I began to get up and come downstairs for a few hours each day. This procedure seemed to help in warding off the nausea which was virtually present all the time and in the expectation of a steady abatement of symptoms, I was anxious not to stay in bed longer than was necessary, thereby avoiding the onset of the flabbiness which is inevitable when one is in bed. It so happened that my doctor was away on holiday during that week and as the course of my illness seemed quite uneventful, I did not call on his partner to visit me and was therefore a law unto myself.

As regards food, this was confined primarily to toast with sweet marmalade, sieved vegetables, a very little lean meat and fruit and salads, all in very small quantity. For my tea every day I used to have a few slices of bread spread with Marmite and slices of tomato. This was the nearest approach to palatable food that I achieved for several weeks. Fat was avoided almost entirely, with the exception of a little milk in tea.

Most of the day I spent sitting quietly in a chair or on a sofa, and the only walking that I did was a maximum of about fifty yards or so in the garden with a walking stick once a day. The above regime continued until June 6th with little change either for the better or the worse. That evening the feeling of nausea intensified quite suddenly and I was unable to eat any supper at all. The next day I lay quietly in bed feeling thoroughly ill and realizing that complete rest in bed was the only possible regime. My diet was very light, virtually fat-free and with very little protein. Toast and marmalade, watery soup and salads and vegetables in small quantity were all that I wanted. The nausea was relieved to some extent by food and the regular consumption of a cup of Bovril and a biscuit half way between breakfast and lunch was a definite help. I also found that grapes were of great assistance and when waves of nausea came over me, two or three grapes helped to ward it off. Although a little food always made me feel better, for the most part I got no pleasure from it whatever except on one or two curious occasions when I suddenly derived real enjoyment from something unusually tasty. Two examples of this were a plateful of young peas straight out of the garden, and on another occasion a helping of bottled shrimps. Both my wife and I had great misgivings as to the possible outcome of this experiment but I got pleasure from it and apparently without the slightest ill effect.

I remained in this condition for a further two weeks during which I steadily lost weight and felt in very poor shape indeed. Apart from the nausea I was permanently afflicted with a taste in my mouth that was both sour and metallic and altogether most unpleasant. In my own estimation I reached rock bottom as regards the severity of the disease almost exactly one month after its commencement. One rather curious thing is that well-meaning enquirers and sympathisers usually referred to the depressing effect of my condition. My own opinion is that the word "depressing" does not accurately describe my feelings. On the whole I was thoroughly fed up with the nausea and the length of time that was elapsing before any indication of an improvement, but I would not say that I was depressed in the sense of a post-influenzal depression. During this period pigmentation of the skin was very marked and reached a maximum, and at the end of the first month I had lost about 2½ stones. The urine was still strongly pigmented but at one month I thought I detected the first sign of a slightly better-coloured stool.

At this stage my doctor indicated that with no real sign of improvement he would like to call in another opinion and I was examined by a surgeon. This examination took place on June 21st and I told the surgeon, quite truthfully, that I thought I was feeling just a little better than I had been a few days previously. Having examined me and taken my case history he and my own doctor both expressed the opinion that they still thought my case was one of straightforward infective hepatitis, but there remained the possibility of obstruction and the need for surgery and he advised my removal to a London hospital for observation, blood tests and surgery if that should prove necessary. I did not welcome the idea of transfer to hospital but could not disagree with the wisdom of taking positive steps to establish a correct diagnosis. The journey to London of twenty miles was accomplished at a fairly slow speed in a comfortable car but, even so, it was a formidable ordeal of a kind that cannot be appreciated by anyone who has not done a longish journey when in very poor shape.

On the first day I was X-rayed with a negative result. Blood tests were taken and I gathered that the blood picture was as expected. During the previous week at home and the first of my two weeks in hospital I was at such a low ebb that I dozed for much of the day and took no interest in the wireless or in reading. During this period I had a slight smarting sensation in the eyes and some degree of aversion to light. Even if I had wanted to read I found any attempt to do so to produce sensations so disagreeable as to be almost painful. Before leaving home I had signed a few cheques in payment of bills and even the effort of signing my name a dozen times left me with a curious sensation of confusion and exhaustion which was probably psychological as much as physical.

The consultant discussed my diet with me and he recommended a low fat regime and a fairly low protein regime pending more positive improvement. Thinking back at this stage I often wonder whether my getting out of bed after about ten days had contributed materially to my relapse and the more severe symptoms of the third, fourth and fifth weeks. I felt instinctively that during the time that I had come downstairs prematurely I did nothing foolish and it is my belief that the illness was going to take the course that it did whether I had stayed in bed or not. Up to now my dietary regime was based on very little of anything and I found it extremely difficult and disagreeable trying to consume what was regarded as an adequate number of soft drinks containing glucose. I cannot help wondering whether it really serves any useful purpose to persuade a patient to drink far more than he instinctively wants. It never seemed to have the slightest effect on my sense of wellbeing or otherwise whether I was drinking a lot or a little. I was also advised to take as much Casilan as possible and endeavoured to take this in Bovril at least once a day. I found it extremely distasteful, however, and felt instinctively that I was not really deriving any worthwhile benefit from it, although I have heard other victims of this complaint say that they took large quantities in various ways apparently without difficulty.

Throughout the first six weeks of the illness I experienced once characteristic and unpleasant symptom. After a period of sleep and during the first few seconds of regaining consciousness, I had a sensation of clear-headedness and well-being. Within a fraction of a second of the return of full consciousness I experienced what seemed to be a surge of contaminated blood to the head which conjured up a mental picture analogous to that of the sea surging into a crevice in the rocks. This sensation of blood-surge was so unpleasant as to amount almost to pain, and at one stage I found myself deliberately trying to avoid dozing off during the day because of the unpleasantness of the experience of awakening. Directly the surge sensation had occurred, all the unpleasant feelings of illness were back again.

The second week in hospital (June 29th) showed the first positive sign of something like an improvement. It happened to be the second week of the Wimbledon Tennis Championships and for the first time I was sufficiently interested in what was going on to listen to the radio. The mere thought of seeing it on the television, however, was quite repugnant to me and I could not watch for more than a second or two. At the same time I was able to start reading a little and sometimes for an hour or two I would almost experience a sense of well-being. From now onwards the usual experience was of ups and downs, with good days and bad days. I was definitely more interested in food and the doctor readily agreed to my having virtually unlimited protein. He still advised very little fat, however, and I had no desire to eat fat. Food that was tasty gave me great pleasure and I particularly enjoyed haddock for breakfast. On one occasion I got round a junior nurse to give me a kipper, which was on the forbidden list but which I am sure did me no harm. During this phase I experienced both desire for and enjoyment of food, but, simultaneously, some degree of nausea. I used to dread meal times and my heart sank at the sight of the tray being brought in, but once I had got over the first few mouthfuls I enjoyed eating and felt better for it.

At the end of the second week further blood tests were taken which indicated a gradual improvement and the doctors agreed to my being sent home (July 6th). At this stage I was eating quite well and for domestic reasons spent the week-end of July 9th—12th at a relative's house a few miles away. Apart from the ten-minute journey by car I was still staying permanently in bed and behaving as an ill patient. In spite of the improving blood picture there was, as yet, no abatement of superficial pigmentation of skin and urine, and only slight improvement in the colour of the stools. On the evening of July 9th I had my last really bad relapse, being unable to eat at all and feeling as bad as at any stage of the illness. This relapse only lasted about twenty-four hours and was all the more unpleasant for coinciding with a heat wave. Thereafter there was a very gradual but continuous improvement and I spent the days lying or sitting on a sofa downstairs, the weather being warm and pleasant.

On July 20th (ninth week) I began to get dressed during the day, took a few steps in the garden and for the first time enjoyed sitting outside in the evening sunshine. Up to then I had tended to have marked photophobia. During the ninth and tenth weeks the skin and urine pigmentation at last began to disappear, taking just about two weeks in the process. Looking upon this time as the beginning of convalescence, a process of very gradual improvement ensued. With improved appetite my weight was on the increase and I felt that I was definitely returning to something like normality. The period of convalescence, which was destined to last from about mid-August until mid-January, was characterized by a continuous but extremely gradual mitigation of all symptoms. The most characteristic and disagreeable remaining symptom was the periodic sensation of bruising and fullness in the central epigastric region. I described this to myself as "bulginess". I found myself adopting a characteristic compensating gait, with rounded shoulders and hollow chest. Occasionally this sensation lasted for a whole day or for several hours during the day, but as time passed the sensation gradually diminished both in length and severity and during the autumn months I would go several days at a time without experiencing it. Occasionally, however, it would return for several hours during the day and I would be virtually unfit for any sort of activity while it lasted. Towards the end of September I first began to take an interest in what had been going on during my illness and with the end of the fine weather about this time, I began to go to work for an hour or two each day.

There is little more to say about the convalescent months except that the periodic return of the sensation of "bulginess" and the occasional experience of near-nausea made it imperative to live from hour to hour and to be prepared to drop everything on the bad days. I am inclined to think that these bad spells were unaffected, either positively or negatively, by physical or mental activity. Sometimes it seemed that mental problems or worries precipitated an attack although on other occasions I found that occupying my mind with something positive helped me to forget my symptoms. During October and November I gradually resumed fairly strenuous forms of physical exercise, notably gardening and Scottish dancing. In spite of the strenuousness of the latter, on no occasion did it ever seem to do me the slightest harm — rather the reverse. The time when I was most likely to feel ill was when sitting quietly, usually before lunch. Almost invariably a meal made me feel better.

Based on my own experience, I am convinced that for a period of several months a convalescent from infective hepatitis should never feel himself obliged to go through with any particular mental or physical activity and should always be prepared to drop everything and rest when instinct tells him to do so. The last occasion on which I felt definitely ill was on the 18th January, 1956, exactly eight months after the start of the illness when an attack of "bulginess" and malaise was brought on by carrying a rather heavy suitcase a matter of several hundred yards. Since that time symptoms have still recurred in very minor degree but have not been sufficient to interfere with any normal activities. I had completely abstained from alcohol up to Christmas when I began taking an occasional small drink of sherry, apparently without the slightest ill effect.

I suggest that the moral from my experience is that in convalescence the patient alone can tell how well or unwell he is and his regime needs to be regulated by his own instincts rather than by any set timetable or rules. I suggest that he will instinctively avoid overdoing it or over-eating, provided that he is always absolutely honest with himself, avoiding the temptation, on the one hand, to malinger and, on the other hand, to force himself to do anything that his instinct tells him is harmful.

Having re-read this account after a gap of 14 years it seems rather naive in parts and medical thought on the treatment of this disease has doubtless changed in that time. There are, however, just one or two after-thoughts I would like to add.

When hepatitis was first diagnosed after about 4 days I was immediately dosed with magnesium sulphate. This I regarded as a barbarous and dubious addition to my other afflictions and I wondered whether it is merely a traditional ritual or whether the benefits conferred justify its use. Secondly, on the question of diet I still believe that the victim is himself the best judge of what is harmful and what is not. Even when nausea was at its height, I occasionally craved for a little of something tasty and appetising. I mentioned potted shrimps as an example and a boiled egg was nearly always acceptable. About the second month I experienced real protein hunger which must surely be indicative of a physiological need. I satisfied this need in the first place by dint of low cunning but a little later with the genuine acquiescence of my doctor. The recovery process was a slow and protracted one. Periodical feelings of malaise became gradually less frequent over a period lasting about 2 years. They were intermittent, usually lasting a few hours perhaps once a week in the earlier stages and once a month as time passed. These attacks seemed to be associated with times of mental stress rather than physical activity. This became quite noticeable and physical activity was even beneficial in aborting an attack. Even now, 14 years later, I very occasionally have mild sensations reminiscent of the earlier phases of the illness and I doubt whether after a really severe attack of hepatitis one is quite the same again. In saying this I would not like unduly to depress a fellow sufferer reading these words since these residual sensations are not sufficient to interfere with one's normal activities apart from awareness that they exist.

On the subject of alcohol I was firmly told not to touch it for six months from recovery. I did, in fact, break this rule discreetly after about three months and as far as subjective sensations were concerned, I never had any reason to suppose that a strictly moderate indulgence did me any harm.

At no time did I have any treatment with drugs other than the magnesium sulphate referred to above.

# Chapter XXIV

# Hyperthyroidism

The important thing about hyperthyroid illness is to recognise it in its early stages, and so avoid the inevitable crash. Recently an airline pilot, working for a famous company, invariably landed his aircraft half an hour before schedule on a fairly short run. He was found to be hyperthyroid. He did everything perfectly but far too fast, and but for an excellent diagnosis many innocent people might have died. The hyperthyroid person is like Badger, of The Wind in the Willows, who dropped out breathless from the Toad Hall Dance muttering, "I can do it for a little, but I can't go on for long". Bouts of hectic activity are followed by periods of intense fatigue, and there is a perfectionist quality about the activity that should alert any physician, when he uses it as a yardstick against the fatigue.

I did not know I was hyperthyroid as mine was a masked case with no eye signs. I had always been very active, but then I tried to walk through an attack of influenza as it was Christmas and there was much to do in the home. I would suddenly become so profoundly tired that all the family noticed it. I would have bouts of activity followed by this incredible fatigue. Everything was an effort and I became restless, anxious, and very depressed because normal household tasks seemed impossible to conclude satisfactorily. I put it all down to a post-influenzal depression; but the fatigue continued. It was not the delightful tiredness after a good days work, but a dreadful lethargy, and a feeling of "all passion spent". There was something most unpleasant about it.

Suddenly I realised I was losing weight rapidly. Over a stone disappeared in eight weeks, although before my weight had been stable for twenty years. I found I was breathless when climbing a small flight of stairs I had previously run up. Social occasions instead of being enjoyable became embarrassing as my heart would race at a rate of knots, and my face would flush the colour of beetroot, and I was conscious of a feeling of excessive warmth. From loving a warm room I craved for a cold one which upset my husband. "You used to be cold in bed, now you are boiling hot and your heart races like a steam engine." My bowels became loose, and the movements diurnal; while in no way approaching diarrhoea there was a change in rhythm which should have alerted me to metabolic change. My eyes were noticed to be very bright. Then when my appetite became eccentric, my emotions labile, and my fatigue profound I at last sought advice; and still the diagnosis eluded me.

The diagnosis was difficult as I was in the throes of an artificial menopause after a vaginal hysterectomy performed eighteen months earlier. This was for menorrhagia and a bad second degree prolapse of the uterus. Domestic problems were prevalent too so a diagnosis of an anxiety state was bandied about; but finally the signs, symptoms and laboratory tests clinched it as a case of hyperthyroidism.

I warned the doctor concerned that I was of the hypersensitive eczema, asthma, migraine, serum sickness type and that I was sensitive to many drugs and chemicals such as penicillin, streptomycin, dettol and many detergents. However, I was treated with 6 microcuries of the isotope $^{131}$I. Everything seemed so simple and straightforward; yet as I drank my cup of isotope I couldn't help thinking of Socrates drinking his hemlock. It all seemed far too easy. It was the calm before the storm. Three months later a tracer test showed I was close to hypothyroidism. Eighteen months later permanent hypothyroidism was proved by another tracer test. Much water flowed under the bridge during that period and I was very ill indeed. Far worse than the illness that had first taken me to hospital — but that is another story.

In autumn 1967 I started to put on weight; it rose gradually from my normal 10st 7lb to 11st.

In January 1968 I had a short, odd illness in which I spent a confused, disorientated night with a feeling of detachment from reality. My temperature was 99° and I attributed it to "flu". It was very frightening.

Thereafter my weight started to fall, and by mid-summer it had fallen to 10st 4lb. During my holiday of 1968 I became aware of increased hunger and restless sleep with early waking — I remember walking beside an Austrian lake at 5 a.m. I often had a sensation of not being 100% conscious and frequently had pain in the small joints of my feet.

During the following autumn and winter my appetite remained noticeably good and I was plagued by insomnia which caused my wife much distress.

Spring 1969 saw difficulty in suturing as I couldn't keep the instruments steady. My writing was deteriorating and I developed a tendency to omit syllables. Patients began to remark that I didn't look well. This was very irritating and I told them I had never felt fitter, which I truly believed.

In summer 1969 I had a three-weeks holiday in France. I ate tremendously, but was unable to sleep without a sedative. I felt much better for half a bottle of wine; it steadied my hand.

Up to this point I had attributed all my symptoms to "nerves" and had pondered the differential diagnosis of neurosis and depression. But when I returned from holiday and found I had lost half a stone in three weeks (9st 6lb), had a resting pulse of 120 and hardly had the strength to mow the lawn I began to think. A holiday had made me more objective and I remembered that my mother, grandfather and aunt had all had thyrotoxicosis. However, I had no goitre or exophthalmos though my buttocks had almost withered away.

I arranged a radioactive iodine uptake which was 60% at four hours with a 48 hour P.B.I.[131] of 5. I started to take Neomercazole, t.d.s., and for two weeks nothing happened. Then during the next two weeks my pulse fell gradually to 80 and my weight started to rise by 4 lb a week. My appetite remained good. My muscles became stronger and I could mow the lawn with ease. I slept well.

On the negative side, I began to experience periods of depression — a feeling of hopelessness and despair. When the influenza epidemic hit us after Christmas I found it very difficult to cope in surgery. I became angry with my treatment and, on my own initiative, I gradually reduced my dose to one tablet b.d.

Then in early February this year I awoke feeling "odd" in the head. I couldn't pin-point any specific pain or other symptom but I was quite convinced that I was dying. My own doctor was summoned and spent an hour reassuring me. I eventually went to sleep, and woke next morning feeling very embarrassed by the whole episode.

I received a lecture on altering my own dose and was put back on two tablets t.d.s. There has been no further trouble. I weigh 11st 7lb and have a normal appetite. They propose to give me a therapeutic dose of radioactive iodine soon.

Looking back, two features of this story interest me. Firstly it took me eighteen months to realise that I was ill, and neither my wife or partner had realised it. Secondly, the most noticeable symptoms were mental. Poor sleep and the feeling of being out of touch with reality were most interesting. I was reminded of the sensation of a large dose of amphetamine when one is very tired. I don't know whether my two episodes of acute disturbance in the night were the result of an upsurge of thyroxine level, but they were both quite terrifying.

# Chapter XXV

# Intervertebral Disc Prolapse

In the warm, dry spring of 1945 I had a heavy fall on the base of the spine, whilst playing hockey. The area was tender and uncomfortable for a week, after which I thought no more of it. A few weeks later, again on the hockey field, I felt a sudden pain in the lumbar spine. This proceeded to a typical attack of lumbago. I did not go off duty but moved about bent for three or four days; within ten days I had recovered completely. At that time I had never heard of intervertebral discs.

During the next two years I had two further attacks of lumbago. Then, after my first game of hockey in the autumn of 1947, I felt a pain down the back of my left leg. This persisted for nine months, during which time I had to give up hockey, though I could play golf. I walked with a limp, and found standing the greatest difficulty. I had no pain at rest, either sitting or in bed. I retained the patellar and ankle reflexes, but had a small area of anaesthesia over the lateral border of the foot and little toe. X-ray of the spine showed no abnormality.

I became free of symptoms by midsummer, and resumed hockey the following season. During the next six years I averaged two attacks of lumbago a year, usually precipitated by playing hockey, which I finally gave up.

In July 1954 my lumbago came on when I lifted a heavy suitcase. I was going to spend three days' holiday in London, followed by a week of strenuous walking and scrambling in the Alps. I spent my time in London walking everywhere I went, stopping at intervals to straighten my back a little more. By the end of the third day I had recovered, and finished my holiday without further symptoms.

My next attack was in February 1955. As this persisted into a third week I persuaded an orthopaedic surgeon to let me have a manipulation by his physiotherapist. This was painful and ineffective; the following night my back "locked" when I turned over in bed, and I had to be removed to hospital by ambulance. After five days resting propped up I was almost symptom-free;

those five days comprise the sole period I have lost from work with this condition.

After this I was supplied with a 16-inch-deep lumbar corset, which I wore for six weeks. I then had another attack of lumbago which made the corset intolerable. As it had not prevented the attack I never wore it again.

For the next six years my attacks of lumbago were less frequent, and ran the normal course of seven to fourteen days. Then, in May 1961 I had a recurrence of pain down the left leg. For the first three days this was not relieved by rest and interfered with sleep. On the third night I took a tablet combining an analgesic with a muscular relaxant. I woke in the night with my left leg completely paralysed and anaesthetic. Power and sensation soon returned after a change of position, but I have never since taken or prescribed such tablets.

By the end of a week my leg was fairly comfortable. I only limped slightly and standing was, again, the greatest difficulty. After a month my symptoms had almost disappeared, but I found that my patellar reflex had gone and I had a small patch of anaesthesia just distal to the patella. These signs lasted for about six months.

Since 1961 my lumbago has been less frequent and less severe, and I have had no further sciatica. My back aches slightly, particularly in cold weather, and it is always stiff on waking. I sometimes have to sit up in bed for half an hour in the early hours of the morning. I have had no further X-rays nor advice on treatment since 1955.

Although I never thought of it for some years, it is clear that the heavy fall in 1945 cracked the outer shell of a disc, without any escape of nucleus pulposus until a few weeks later — a not unusual history. The first attack of sciatica was from the fifth lumbar disc and that in 1961 from the third lumbar, an uncommon site, but indisputable from the signs.

I attach no importance to negative X-ray findings in the disc syndrome, unless a myelogram has been performed, a drastic procedure which I would only accept when operation appeared to be indicated. Disc trouble is not supposed to lead to arthritis, but my back is now giving a fair imitation of this. There is no clinical indication for a further X-ray to satisfy scientific curiosity.

It may be that prolapsed intervertebral discs appear to have become much commoner during the past twenty-five years because they are treated more seriously and therefore wrongly. I am quite sure that the important principle in treatment of an established disc lesion is mobility at all times. I concede that a first attack in a young man may demand rest in bed followed by immobilization in plaster, in the hope that healing may take place, but once it is certain that the disc will not recover, to stiffen the spine and weaken its muscles with restrictive corsets is unnatural and wrong. I have never understood how a manipulation should induce extruded disc tissue to return to its place between the vertebrae, nor have I heard or read any explanation of this on anatomical lines by its exponents. Similarly, I have never seen any useful result from formal physiotherapy. My belief is that the normal movements of the body and back will correct the extrusion in the minimal time. My experience of "walking off" lumbago in three days confirms this belief; unfortunately I have only once had the time to devote to this method.

Orthopaedic surgeons constantly exhort their disc patients not to dig their gardens or lift heavy weights. I have continued to do both, even actually during an attack of lumbago, with absolute impunity. I admit that I am always very carcful to bend my knees rather than my back, and to avoid sudden jerks and twists with the back bent. In golf I found putting a great deal more difficult than driving; similarly, in the garden, I find grass-edging the most tiresome operation, because of the slightly bent posture.

I am very glad that I declined an offer of operation when I had my first sciatica in 1947. It would not have prevented the involvement of the third disc in 1961.

I have been very fortunate that my sciatica only caused pain at rest for one short period, but I attribute this partly to my insistence on maintaining normal mobility. I agree that a persistence of sciatic pain at rest is an indication for traction, or for operation in suitable cases, but never for a spinal corset.

# Chapter XXVI

# Keratosis of the Scalp

This story begins with a road accident. I was passenger in the front seat of a car which, entering from a side street, was out of control and dashed across the road into a bank. When it was half way across, my brain was perfectly clear. I realised that the accident was bound to happen. A second later I was still sitting as before but my head was beginning to pour with blood and there was a big hole in the windscreen, through which it had passed. I had no recollection whatever of the accident though my brain was quite clear. I would not have imagined such a clearly cut period of amnesia with my memory perfect before and after.

The wounds in the scalp necessitated the insertion of more than twenty silkworm gut stitches, and all healed by first intention. When the stitches were removed, my scalp was "lumpy" and I could clearly detect at least one hard crust in the exact line of a scar. This crust remained and others gradually appeared during the next few years.

For many years before the accident I had been troubled with dandruff. It became troublesome now and then, and my scalp would feel as if full of buzzing bees. I felt as if I had my cap on. Treatment with a simple ointment for three weeks would restore it to comfort for some months. During the years after the accident the crusts increased in number to more than a dozen, all in the area of the scars. In addition during the fifth year my forehead came to look as if it had been blistered by a tropical sun, covered by a densely adherent scurf. It was not very troublesome, though it itched frequently, but was slowly spreading and was becoming disfiguring. Ointments, old and modern, proved useless, so my doctor and I sought expert advice. The dermatologist diagnosed the condition as keratosis, and stated it was incurable.

I accepted his opinion without surprise or dismay. But after six weeks I suddenly revolted and on impulse took action. I started with soap and water and vigorous massage for an hour. Next day I got a dandruff shampoo (The Classic) and used this every morning for a fortnight. The scurf of my forehead slowly yielded. It was densely adherent. I diminished the frequency of shampooing after a fortnight. By a month the improvement was manifest. The crusts were firmly adherent, and incorporated with the scalp tissue. I used my finger nail as curette and their partial removal caused bleeding. The larger ones would be the size of a finger nail. About the sixth day I noticed a peculiar occurence. In the line of a scar were two drops of fluid. Each had oozed through a hole in the scar. It was oily fluid and in cooling solidified and formed a crust. Half an hour after a shampoo my scalp felt covered with these hard bristles.

This confirmed the opinion I had formed that at the time of the accident, the infection that caused the dandruff, hitherto confined to the sebaceous glands, had been diffused through the tissues of the scalp. It was an oily seborrhoea. In places the manufacture of oil was sufficient to maintain a hole and so a crust was formed. Where there was no hole, it oozed through the skin and became firmly adherent scurf.

Later on that excellent book, Savill's Diseases of the Scalp (1962 edition) came into my hands. The paragraphs relating to keratosis were vague and unsatisfactory, but for this variety of seborrhoea, its recommendation was very definite — massage of the scalp, timed by the clock, prolonged each sitting, and persevering — just what I had been doing. There was no doubt that the massage emptied the scalp of the oily fluid, which would be replaced by a more healthy liquid.

Under this treatment the keratotic crusts slowly diminished in number, so slowly that my barber would not concede *any* improvement for some months. By six months the remaining crusts were firm, and these proved very obstinate. Now, eighteen months have passed since treatment was begun. All the crusts have gone, all scurf has gone, and no ordinary observer would detect any abnormality. It is a great relief. But I no longer neglect paying due attention to the care of my scalp.

# Chapter XXVII

# Migraine

Much has been written about migraine being hereditary, often alternating with epilepsy, and for this reason I have to mention the nocturnal grand mal seizures of my late mother and the occasional scotomata of both my sisters.

My mother had a pronounced aversion from unpleasant noises; she was really horrified by a creaking door, a knife scratching on the plate or by the speech impediment of a stutterer, lest such acoustic irritants might induce an attack that she was dreading all the time. Was she reminded of her own sinister outcry which preceded her seizures? I shall keep this acoustic effect in mind until later on, when I shall describe its optic equivalent in migraine.

My personality corresponds more or less to the classic description of the migraine sufferer, being of an "anxious, striving, perfectionistic, order-loving, rigid" character.

My attacks always start suddenly, and invariably with optic phenomena. First come scintillating scotomata which brings with them immediately the horrible realization that this might be the beginning of a 24-hour period of suffering, when all activities come to a standstill. There are still some minutes of grace which can be utilized for bringing oneself to safety from traffic, for cancelling an appointment or informing the wife of the impending calamity.

Not much time is left: soon the scotoma develops into turning cog-wheels, fortification spectra and hemianopsia. This is the moment when the side of the subsequent headache can be predicted: the left hemianopsia augurs a right hemicrania and vice versa.

There is still a faint hope that all this might abortively come to a stop without developing into a full-scale attack; otherwise the following stations of passion appear: paraesthesiae — ipsilaterally to the previously described hemianopsia — of the fingers, beginning at the thumb and affecting each of the others in turn up to the last one, together with paraesthesiae of the tongue on the corresponding side.

I am coming now to another symptom which I have never seen mentioned in published reports, or heard of from fellow sufferers: "physiognomic amnesia", the inability during the attack to recall faces of people. Even relatives and friends leave a complete blank in my mind if I try to visualize their facial characteristics. This symptom is a constant feature in my attacks, irrespective of whether headache is on the right or on the left side. There are no other losses of memory during the attack: melodies, numbers, rooms, and streets, for instance, can always be recalled without difficulty.

The speech-centre is always involved, when the seizure is situated in the left hemisphere, with resulting aphasia-paraphasia, alexia and inability to comprehend the speech of others. It is indeed a very depressing and frightening experience to be so isolated from near and dear ones, even if one realizes by logical reasoning that this handicap is' of short duration only.

And, indeed, we soon come to the second part of the attack, which consists of unilateral headache, nausea and vomiting, lasting up to 24 hours.

Such seizures may occur some 3-4 times a year, which sounds perhaps reasonable and tolerable, considering the attack-free on the other 361 days of the year. But this unfortunately is not so. These other days may be free of attacks; however, they are certainly not free from worrying and expecting the next scotoma any moment, considering Murphy's Law: "If anything can go wrong, it will — and at the worst possible time.".

Because of this permanent uncertainty I am always reluctant to fix a date for an appointment, to promise my appearance at a meeting, or to take upon myself to deliver a lecture. This also might have influenced my professional choice of radiotherapy: every form of surgical activity would have been contraindicated by my migrainous sword of Damocles, not knowing when it will strike and for what reason.

Of course, about the reason or, perhaps better, the initiating factor nothing definite is known. My chance of having an attack in a hotel during holidays seems to be bigger than in an everyday setting.

Meteorological influences are often claimed by migraine sufferers, particularly in "Chamsin"-weather. This is an eastern wind from the desert, especially in spring and autumn, characterised by dryness and high temperature, being more or less the Israel variety of the "Foehn" in Bavaria and Switzerland, or the "Mistral" in the South of France.

But the principal inducing factor of my attacks seems to consist of optical impressions. If I mentioned at the beginning the "acoustic effect" on an epileptic personality, it is the optic equivalent in my case. If the former might be called "phonophobia", the latter would be "photophobia" in its strictest meaning repugnance towards electric light bulbs without lampshade, to light glaring from a shiny metallic surface, or sunrays reflected from the wind-shield of an oncoming car. Such things give me the "fear" of an impending attack, perhaps only because of the similarity of this eye-strain with the so-dreaded scotoma.

My interest in prophylactic treatment has always been rather limited, considering the timing of my attacks. It never appealed to me particularly to take pills all the year round, hoping that such treatment might be successful and decrease the incidence from 3-4 to 2-3 attacks yearly. I once tried Luminal for many months, although without any appreciable benefit.

Of course, I often took ergotamine at the scotoma stage with the intention of stopping further developments, but such experiments were always inconclusive: seizures may progress to the full-scale affair, or stop in the beginning stage, irrespective of ergotamine being taken or not.

My attitude towards treatment is best expressed by the following rule of thumb. If the headache is somehow tolerable and not of too long duration I just stick it out. Otherwise: 0.01—0.015 mg of morphine subcutaneously stops every attack in minutes, and this is the last refuge which, fortunately, has not been habit-forming in my case.

With advancing age, migraine attacks usually cease to appear. I am at present 61 years old, and my migraine is still going strong.


I suppose my history of migraine dates from my early childhood although I was aware of it only as severe headache at the time. Then, as now, the headaches were mainly on one side of the head, in either temple or in the front of the forehead. They were severe and long lasting, often for most of a day. My mother used to rub the sore head or apply pressure with the palms of her hands which used to afford relief.

In my family, my mother, a sister and 2 brothers, of a total of 8 siblings, have suffered incapacitating headaches, almost certainly migraine.

During adolescence and youth my migraine was not so noticeable. My years as a medical student were apparently free of severe migraine. A severer phase of my migraine has been associated with a more active career since taking up a university and consultant appointment.

Certain background factors, appear consistently with attacks of migraine in my experience. Of these I am aware of physical fatigue from insufficient or disturbed sleep and mental stress or pressurising situations involved in the detail of a daily schedule and also in interpersonal relationships, as precipitants of migraine. The partaking of alcohol, which I enjoy drinking socially at ordinary times, is likely to precipitate a migraine attack in the situations I have cited.

A generalised dull feeling, sometimes a sense of lethargy on starting the day is a frequent warning of a migraine day. Frequently it is a vague abdominal discomfort accompanied by a sensation of incomplete bowel evacuation or even true constipation at the beginning of a hurried day. I have noticed that a state of irritability during the course of a trying day frequently precedes a migraine. If I miss a meal, especially lunch, I have noticed a susceptibility to migraine that day.

At the start of a migraine attack and often throughout it I notice certain visual disturbances. It may be double vision, blurring of the vision or areas of blindness in one eye. I first took notice of the blind patches when I found I could not read print except by covering the affected eye with the hand. At other times I have noticed an involuntary fluttering sensation in the eyelids. Several times I have been aware of shadows, I suppose partially blind patches, in one eye. I remember an eerie sensation walking along a street pavement seeing such a shadow moving forward as I walked. When I have tried to lie down, as I find myself wanting to do, I have seen flickering splashes of colour, usually purple, sometimes scarlet or green, crossing the darkness of my closed eyes.

The typical migraine headache begins with a dull, localised ache which develops rapidly, usually over less than half an hour, into a severe, throbbing headache often of bursting character, deeply seated and relentless, lasting anything from 4 hours to a whole day and night, often longer. Sometimes I feel a deep, boring soreness in the eyeball and orbit on the affected side. The eyeball feels tender to touch and when I touch my head or attempt to comb my hair the affected side of the head feels numb and sore. A loss of appetite and nausea are invariable accompaniments. I have frequently had retching and vomiting which has not necessarily relieved the migraine attack.

There is variation in the severity of the attacks. On the average, I have had anything from one to 4 attacks per week. Frequently,

I have had migraine each successive day for 3 and 4 day periods
with relief lasting several weeks. At times of leave from ordinary
duties the attacks have definitely lessened in frequency and
severity but one of the worst attacks I ever experienced occurred
after an air journey during a leave with less than 5 hours of sleep
the night before and obligatory socialising after arrival at my
destination. That time I was knocked out by severe migraine for
nearly 18 hours and I was quite unable to lie down because of
continuous bursting pain. I have also suffered migraine over
weekends on a Sunday when stress factors, to all intents and
purposes, are lacking. Similar attacks have occurred at the
beginning of a planned leave. Presumably the change from
routine has been the triggering mechanism. Explosive attacks of
migraine have sometimes woken me up from fitful sleep and
remained with me for most of the following day.

The exasperating feature of the migraine attack is the inability
to get on with my work. That which is achieved during a mild
attack is often ineffective. Straightforward everyday activity
such as making hospital rounds and driving a car can be a strain
and effort.

When I am conscious of the onset of an attack I take a 5 gr
tablet of aspirin together with a 1 mg tablet of ergotamine and
caffeine (Migril) in the belief that I shall minimise the attack
but I am not convinced of the efficacy of this regime. Usually
nothing seems to touch a full-blown attack. I have tried ordinary
aspirin which I find irritating to the stomach, producing a feeling
of soreness in the epigastrium which itself might be a migraine
equivalent. I have tried codeine compounds but I do not like
them because of the abdominal distention and constipation
which I have suffered as result of the medication. More than anything, I have found it relieving to lie down, curled up, the
curtains drawn with the head buried against a pillow. I have found
diazepam tablets (Valium) 2.5 to 5 mg helpful in sleeping off a
migraine attack. The relief of a normal-feeling head on waking
up after a severe attack of migraine can only be likened to the
becalming effect of a lull after a terrible storm.

I suppose the adjustments I am trying to make in my work
will help reduce the frustrations and anxieties and make my
migraine more tolerable. I have reached the age of wearing reading glasses which I imagine will ease the strain on my eyes.
Advancing years in any case has brought me better insight into
the psychological factors.

I am aware of another kind of transient headache I have had
in stress situations. The feeling is like that of a tight band around

the head. It is usually not severe and I regard it as a tension headache distinct from a migraine headache.

I have discussed my migraine with a neurologist, himself a
migraine sufferer, and I am convinced that I do not want any
special investigations carried out. I feel also that while psychiatric
advice might help control my migraine I understand myself
sufficiently well in a semi-objective way not to want to seek it. I
am aware that I possess an obsessional temperament. I suppose
it is some consolation to know that several professional colleagues
I know well also suffer severe forms of migraine but presumably
continue to lead active and satisfying lives.


I have never seen an adequate description of migraine in any
textbook. My right to describe a classical attack has been thrust
upon me because I have suffered more than a thousand severe
migraine attacks spanning a period of forty five years. On May
8th, 1968, I had a sub-total adrenalectomy performed for hypertension, electrolyte disturbance, and excess of aldosterone.
Bilateral hyperplasia was found in the glands. Since then I have
had NO MIGRAINE so I hope I can write objectively as a cured
case.

History is important in migraine so I must give the background.
I grew up with migraine. It was a much feared household word.
As a small child I remember my mother withdrawing to her room
from time to time apparently dying, her face the colour of the
Cliffs of Dover, her eyes agonised with pain, utterly prostrate,
retching and being sick every twenty minutes for an interminable
twelve hours. It seemed impossible that one so ill could live. Next
day she would appear looking bonnier than ever, with bright
alert eyes, and a rosy face, just as if nothing had happened. It
was uncanny. At the age of seventy eight she died very suddenly
during an attack of migraine, with much sickness and muscle
weakness. Apart from migraine she had had no illness of note
all her life. In that moment of time she wrecked effectively two
common textbook statements that it is an illness you grow out
of, and no one ever dies of the disease.

Her post mortem showed a dissecting aneurysm of the aorta
caused by a large haematoma weakening the wall, the haematoma
perhaps caused by the retching and struggling with sickness for
many years, huddling in an unnatural position over a vomit bowl.

Whereas sickness was the dominant feature of my mother's
attacks, headache was my most serious symptom. The pattern of

my many attacks was fairly constant, twice a month like clock-
work.

I would crawl into bed the previous evening feeling tired and
not my gay self, so I thought a period must be on its way. Then
about five next morning I would wake suddenly feeling drugged
and dazed as if I had been in a deep, restless sleep all night. It
was just as if an air raid siren had given its warning note, or I was
on a troopship again and the action stations bell had just rung
the alarm. There was an impending sense of doom, panic stations
personified, and great anxiety and restlessness. It was difficult
opening my eyes as the eyelids seemed feeble and sluggish, and
when I had opened them I wished I hadn't as the horrible headache was there. It always started over my dominant left eye, then
passed like a thunderbolt through my left eyeball, a throbbing,
boring, brutal pain that made me feel desperately sick. This area
was my Achilles heel at first; so as a small child, not knowing
quite what had hit me, I told my mother "I've got a corner of
a headache".

It was an apt description but it was no hole and corner affair
for within an hour half the head was involved, and the headache
would work up to a great crescendo for twelve endless hours and
eventually the whole head was throbbing, and cracking in all
directions. The head hurt to touch and was tender all over. Sometimes a spontaneous black eye would occur, and odd bruises
appear on the limbs. My hair was always unruly, and in a bad
attack would stand up like a cat's tail in a quarrel. I could never
get warm in bed however many blankets and hot water bottles
I had — my hands and feet remained persistently cold with a
blanched, ischaemic look. During most of the attack my heart
would slow to fifty, my breathing become shallow, my blood
pressure be raised (210/120 on several occasions instead of its
normal 140/90) and most of my sphincters remained obstinately
closed so that it was impossible to pass faeces or urine, and the
sickness that often occurred was usually the most horrible endless
retching that nearly tore the gut out. Polyuria and a real bout of
sickness heralded the end of the attack. Food and drink were
abhorrent until afterwards, when the odd thing was that anything
could be eaten with no discomfort at all.

In a bad attack with much retching the colon would go into
spasm, and there was muscle weakness too so that if I was up and
about climbing stairs and struggling into clothes became an ordeal.
The one hope was that in time the attack would pass and a wonderful feeling of warmth and well being would flood in with polyuria,
and tachycardia, and an enormous appetite, and no more pain.

Migraine is one of the less desirable hereditary acquisitions. It has affected my mother, myself and one of my daughters. I had my first attack about the age of fifteen when at school and can remember the novel effect of teichopsia upon Greek prose which I was endeavouring to translate. I had very few attacks during my university years but their frequency increased during hospital training and subsequent consultant work. I suppose I have averaged one attack a fortnight up to my present age of sixty except when on holidays. During the forty-five years the pattern of the attacks has not changed, although I think I have fewer severe ones, possibly because of prophylactic measures. Most of the attacks are mild and only of nuisance value, a fair number are moderately severe and significantly inconvenient and a few, perhaps six in a year, are very severe and totally incapacitating. Although the average occurrence of attacks is about one a fortnight — frequently at weekends — I also get occasional "clusters" of mild attacks during four or five consecutive days.

Although I have come to recognize certain provocative factors which are almost always followed by an attack, the majority of attacks are unpredictable and have no obvious trigger. I think it is important for sufferers from migraine to recognize any provocative factors, particularly those which precede severe attacks, because appropriate measures may modify or prevent the attack. In my own case I recognize from bitter experience the unwise but frequently unavoidable pastime of "clock-chasing". This means non-stop intellectual activity and anxiety entailed by an unusual spate of professional work and responsibility, mixed up with meetings, social events, domestic obligations and "things that can't wait" for three or four days running. In spite of the high-pressure existence nothing happens until things ease up, and then a severe attack of migraine takes place. A variant of this is the "ordeal", namely some important professional or social event which causes me anxiety and apprehension for days beforehand because no failure in personal performance or punctuality can be allowed. In the event everything goes off all right but a severe attack of migraine often follows. Foodstuffs which provoke my attacks — usually mild ones — are of high residue type. Thus porridge for breakfast on two or more days running will always do it, as well as fruit consisting mostly of pips and skin such as gooseberries and currants, and their derivatives in the form of jam, fruitcake and Christmas pudding. Black currants are peculiarly noxious in that I do not necessarily need to eat them because their aroma when my wife is making jelly or the smell of the bushes when I am picking the fruit, will often give me a mild attack. I am quite sure that alcohol *per se* does not provoke my migraine but what undoubtedly can do so are the circumstances and environment in which it is taken. Thus I can have a couple of drinks before dinner and half-a-bottle of wine with the meal with impunity. But far less alcohol taken at a noisy cocktail party in a smoke-laden atmosphere at the end of a busy day may well give me a severe migraine next morning. Similarly a few glasses of champagne at a wedding do me good but if I take just one glass to assist me proposing the bride's health I get a migraine that evening. But here I think the "ordeal" mechanism is responsible.

The pattern of my attacks may be mild, moderately severe or very severe. Mild attacks consist of visual disturbance alone or a mild unilateral headache which usually occurs alone but occasionally follows the visual disturbance. They start suddenly at any time. The visual disturbances are classical. I suddenly become aware of a small shimmering scotoma in the centre of my field of vision which upsets a person's face, a line of print or whatever I am looking at. Peripheral vision is unaffected at this stage. The central scotoma persists for about five minutes and then slowly enlarges. As it does so the central shimmering expands to its periphery and develops there into a zone of scintillating zig-zag flashes of white light or teichopsia. Vision returns to the central part of the field of vision as the teichopsia moves out centrifugally in a crossed hemianopic or, rarely, quadrantic manner. As the teichopsia progresses outwards it increases in amplitude and becomes coloured, mostly yellow, red, green and blue, to form the classical fortification spectra. The process continues with return of vision behind the advancing fortification spectra until the latter pass out of the visual fields. The duration of the visual phenomena is about twenty-five minutes from start to finish. Both eyes are affected but the signs are usually more vivid in one eye and their distribution is not always strictly hemianopic. Unless a headache follows clearing of the eyesigns I feel perfectly all right although on a very few occasions a second attack of the visual disturbances has followed shortly after the first.

If a headache follows the eyesigns or starts by itself *de novo* I become aware of it in the supraorbital and temporal areas on one side. I have never noticed any undue pulsation in the temporal artery; compression of it does not improve or alter the headache nor does release of compression increase it. The quality of the headache is dull, non-pulsatile, mild and uninfluenced by bending down or head movements. It is a nuisance but does not

interfere with my work. I am slightly off my food and notice
some unusual belching and heartburn. Sometimes I get vague
abdominal pain which I interpret as colon spasm since it is
relieved by the passage of small scyballous faeces. The other
characteristic accompaniment of the mild headache is yawning.
As a rule the headache lasts for the rest of the day but has gone
by next morning.

Moderately severe attacks are more troublesome because they
impair my intellectual ability and capacity for decisive action.
As a rule I have no premonitory visual disturbance but become
aware of a dull headache during the course of the morning. It is
more generalized than that of mild attacks but more intense and
tends to get worse as the day goes on. I find myself becoming
rather vague and indecisive with difficulty in planning the stages
of investigation or regime of treatment in a complicated case.
My writing deteriorates in quality and spelling mistakes are
frequent. I also become slightly dysphasic to the extent of
difficulty in finding the right word in conversation or writing.
These obvious cortical symptoms are difficult to describe
adequately and even more so to analyse. It seems that the
faculty of assembling and coordinating information and acting
upon it in the form of verbal instructions is impaired and that a
similar incoordination affects speech and writing. For instance,
the spelling mistakes and deterioration in quality of my writing
are due to real dysgraphia and poor formation of the correct
letters rather than the use of incorrect ones. This process tends
to get worse as the day goes on and I stop work simply because
I know that I am not fit to cope with any tricky situation. I also
feel slightly nauseated and may vomit if I eat anything although
I can tolerate liquids. I find that I feel generally incompetent
mentally and just want to go home to bed. Although I yawn
repeatedly I am not bodily tired but just find it increasingly
difficult to produce the mental stimulus for physical activity.

My very severe attacks are quite overwhelming and totally
incapacitating. They are characterized by persistent vomiting
and retching accompanied by inability to make any significant
mental effort. They always start in the early morning, waking
me up about 5.0 or 6.0 a.m. with a severe, dull, generalized
headache which is increased by any movement of the head. It is
not pulsatile or "bursting" but is worst in the frontal and
temporal areas. It is accompanied by vasomotor disturbances in
which coldness to the point of goose-flesh and shivering lasting
three to four minutes, alternates with vasodilatation and sweating — especially on the face and neck — for the same duration. I

am restless and feel indescribably wretched and ill. After about twenty minutes of these initial symptoms waves of nausea begin with increasing gastric peristalsis and vomiting begins. The effort of getting rapidly to the lavatory makes the headache and other symptoms worse still. The initial vomit is enormous; the previous evening's dinner returns apparently quite undigested and recognizable. It seems that my stomach must have been atonic and devoid of digestive function for some twelve hours.

The strain of vomiting accentuates the headache and vasomotor disturbance and I stumble back to bed shivering, pale and haggard and literally willing to die. For the next two or three hours the dismal process is repeated with ataxic journeys to the lavatory every quarter-of-an-hour or so although vomiting is replaced by the retching of mucus and bile. Headache and vasomotor instability continue and prostration is complete. Any consecutive thought or mental activity is in abeyance and photophobia is intense. Gradually the intervals between retching lengthen and snatches of sleep become possible. By the afternoon the headache is better, the vasomotor symptoms have ceased, but the nausea remains and the only mental activity appears to be a desire for further sleep. In the early evening there is a decided improvement and the headache has gone. When I get out of bed I am still shaky and ataxic, vague and dysphasic and quite incapable of sustained conversation or answering the telephone. I am also ketotic and thirsty and can tolerate small quantities of iced tonic water. But anorexia persists and the thought of food or smell of cooking is almost intolerable. I do not care what the time is but just want more sleep. The usual washing and teeth-cleaning formalities require a mental effort instead of being automatic.

The next day I am a good deal better physically and am able to get up at the usual time. But I am still ketotic and shaky and find that the processes of shaving and dressing require deliberate thought instead of automatic action. I can manage a light breakfast but I cannot read the newspaper without considerable effort and I know that I could not undertake a ward round or outpatient clinic. I am still vague and somewhat dysphasic and writing remains uncertain. I usually sit about in the house and go off to sleep again as there is really nothing that I can do which requires no mental effort. But after lunch I am usually well enough to go outside for a walk or go up to the hospital and hear what has gone on in my absence. The next day I have quite recovered.

So far as treatment is concerned, I try and avoid the provocative factors mentioned above. But, human nature being what it is and various professional and social obligations being inescapable, I am not always successful. When I recognize that I am in for a spell of "clock-chasing" or have a prospective "ordeal" I sometimes take Valium or phenobarbitone for several days but it is hard to assess their value. They certainly do not prevent some severe attacks from taking place but, equally, I do not invariably have one if I fail to take the drugs.

For the attacks themselves the mild ones need no treatment, but for moderately severe attacks any of the tablets containing ergotamine tartrate, such as Cafergot or Migril are of definite value provided that they are taken as early in the attacks as possible. They do not abort or stop moderately severe attacks but they do modify them and prevent them getting worse and usually enable me to finish a day's work.

For very severe attacks no oral treatment can be effective because of the persistent vomiting. I have tried tablets of ergotamine tartrate sublingually but gave them up years ago because their unpleasant taste just hastened the onset of vomiting. Nor could I possibly summon up the mental or physical resources needed for preparing and giving myself an injection of ergotamine tartrate.

The only treatment which I find possible, and which is conspicuously beneficial, is the use of Cafergot suppositories. I keep some in the bedside cupboard and insert one as soon as I awake with a severe attack. They do not act quickly enough to prevent the first one or two vomits but, because they contain a barbiturate, they put me off to sleep and save me hours of misery. As a rule I wake up again after four or five hours relatively well. I can eat a light breakfast, I have no headache, but I am slightly dysphasic and indecisive. However, I can manage the day's work and by midday am pretty well normal. There is no doubt whatever that Cafergot suppositories have made an immense difference to my life and it is remarkable that their use is not mentioned in the standard textbooks.

Migraine headache has been known for at least 3500 years. A papyrus discovered in the tomb of Thebes includes a description of a "sickness of half the head". In the first century A.D. Aretaeus of Cappadocia described a paroxysmal, one-sided, severe head pain associated with nausea. Galen in the second century introduced the word hemicrania which was gradually modified into the present-day term of migraine.

There are numerous reports on migraine written by physicians who have personally experienced the characteristic syndrome. Many of these appeared in the neurologic literature of the late 19th and early 20th century. I should like to present here my personal experience coupled with some of the more recent advances in the psychology and physiology of the migraine syndrome.

My interest in migraine became intense several years ago when I experienced a rather abrupt onset of frequent severe headaches. Prior to that time I had not considered myself to be a migraine sufferer. But as with many medical experiences, a retrospective analysis uncovered evidence to the contrary. Later I shall discuss in detail the various trigger mechanisms in migraine headache but will mention here that even as a child I became aware of certain facts related to the production of severe headaches associated with nausea. I learned that prolonged periods in intense sunlight could result in headache. Even though I was somewhat protected from this phenomenon in New York City where I lived for most of my life, each summer I worked on an uncle's farm where sunshine was abundant and long days were spent working in open fields. I remember the regular occurrence of severe headaches each evening until I learned that the use of a protective cap to shield my eyes from sunlight completely eliminated the difficulty. I also became aware of the relationship between a prolonged unnatural visual stimulus and migraine, finding that headaches regularly followed attendance at a movie. Early in childhood I learned to take salicylates before going to a movie in order to avoid the inevitable consequence of an afternoons's enjoyment.

Although I can trace the onset of migraine headaches to my childhood, they were not sufficiently frequent or severe to interfere with normal activity. The abrupt increase which I experienced several years ago I attribute to a greater liability of blood pressure and vasomotor activity with increasing age. This lability of vasomotor activity as influenced by environmental agents (pharmacological or psychological) I feel is related to the production of the migraine headache.

From a personal view it is difficult to provide an unbiased description of the migraine personality. Nevertheless, certain features are sufficiently characteristic that they are recognized by most of the individuals suffering from migraine. Indeed, in reading the description of the migraine personality by H. G. Wolff in "Headache and Other Head Pain", I could not help but feel that it was a personal account.

A constant feature is a mood of compulsiveness which dominates daily existence. The compulsiveness may pervade all activities or may be limited to several specific areas. During my childhood I remember redoing drawings, painting, and other projects because of small imperfections. There was also a desire for orderliness. Toys and books all had a proper place and were always put back at the end of the day. I was rarely disciplined about the appearance of my room because it was always kept in order. In college I was terribly bothered by a roommate who took as much pride in disorder as I did in order. As I became older the desire for orderliness led to the use of file systems, indexed notebooks, and almost any system which would prevent disarray of thought or form.

The compulsive trait frequently leads to a great deal of frustration. This is particularly true when something must be left undone as an uncompleted task is in a sense a form of imperfection. During the first year of medical school I had great difficulty in bringing myself to realize that I could not learn every detail of medical subjects. I remember studying the voluminous Gray's "Anatomy" attempting to memorize each fine anatomical point. Frustration and disappointment resulted when I realized that it was an impossibility.

The two traits of compulsiveness and perfectionism are not necessarily derived from external pressures but from internal drives. The individual with a migraine personality is, therefore, usually a conscientious workman and the performance of his occupation is carried out with skill and with little need of supervision. Because of these features, the individual is frequently given a great deal of responsibility even during childhood. In most instances these attributes would appear to be desirable. In extreme cases, however, the internal drive leads to an interference of overall performance. There might, for example, be a reluctance to take on new tasks before completing tasks on hand. Frequently there is a reluctance to permit someone else to perform a particular task. In the everyday practice of medicine I found myself in a conflict between a desire to take a complete history and perform a physical examination on all patients on one hand and a crowded waiting room on the other. For the individual with a migraine propensity who cannot escape such a dilemna, an increased frequency of migraine headaches results. In my case, the dilemma was solved by a gravitation toward academic medicine where the patient load was smaller, where patients could be examined in detail, and where the day could be arranged with a great deal more organization. The greatest frequency of migraine headaches was experienced during a two-year period in the army. There I found not only a conflict of philosophies but also found it necessary to examine an excessive number of patients in a manner which I felt was entirely inadequate. An additional feature of the migraine personality, obstinacy, increased the conflict. The immovable military outlook frequently collided with my immovable philosophies. The psychological conflict generated in those circumstances caused continuous daily tension with frequent migraines.

During my military experience migraine occurred on an average three to four times a week compared to one or two every six months at present. I gained my greatest experience of the details of migraine during that period. I soon became adept at recognizing the subtle factors which influence the development of the migraine headache. I was able not only to diagnose the varied forms of migraine but also to recognize some of the unusual presentations in very young children. I became sufficiently adept at recognizing the patients suffering from migraine that I could recognize them in the waiting room prior to hearing or seeing their complaints. The pale complexion, squinted eyes, dilated temporal blood vessels, and stiff posture which protected against sudden movement were characteristic features.

The features of the migraine personality have been presented in detail as an understanding of this aspect is necessary if one is to help an individual to reduce the frequency of attacks. The patient must realize that perfectionist and compulsive traits when thwarted result in frustration and inner turmoil. The psychological events are translated into physiological responses and the headache begins. Periods of intense productivity may lead to similar physiological responses in the absence of frustration. After relaxation, both physical and mental, the prodromal symptoms appear — scotomata, flashing lights, double vision, blurring of vision. The headache may follow the prodrome rapidly or develop slowly.

Although some patients may deny the existence of the prodrome, I found that it almost always occurs and can be defined for each individual once they are given the details of the different forms. I have found, for example, that some individuals may not have visual prodromes but may experience vague feelings of depression or oppression and occasionally of euphoria. Personally, I have found that the prodrome may begin as feelings of intense productivity with an unwillingness to retire. It is important for the physician to help the patient elicit the symptoms of the prodrome as it is only during this period that the migraine headache can be completely prevented.

As the migraine headache usually occurs after physical and mental relaxation, one might anticipate that the patient might awaken in the early morning hours with a full-blown headache. This is, indeed, common; however, during periods of continuous activity with little rest or sleep, the headache may occur after "catch-up" sleep. Individuals with migraines frequently talk about "weekend" headaches for the same reason. I found Sunday morning particularly hazardous in this regard. On this morning there is no alarm to awaken me. A leisurely breakfast is followed by attendance in a church with comfortable pews and if the sermon is reassuring rather than controversial, a migraine is certain to follow.

The first day of vacation seems also to be associated with the development of a migraine. In these circumstances, however, I found that relaxation was not entirely to blame. Vacations are usually spent in hotels where a late breakfast is the rule. During the work week breakfast is early and a cup of coffee is always consumed. Over the years I have gained the impression that withdrawal of caffeine can precipitate a migraine headache. The caffeine withdrawal headache is well documented even among normal individuals. Breakfast and coffee during vacation are usually taken late and perhaps this allows sufficient time to elapse to permit escape from the chronic vasoconstrictive effect of caffeine. The end result is vasodilatation and migraine.

The intensity of a migraine headache appears to be directly related to the intensity of the stimulus resulting in vasoconstriction and the rapidity with which the stimulus is dissipated. Rapid vasoconstriction followed by rapid vasodilatation results in severe headache which is virtually impossible to prevent. In my own experience, this sequence occurs most frequently when I am required to give a research paper or to speak before a large audience. I find myself relatively relaxed until the few moments before I am about to speak. Then tachycardia begins and the pulse becomes stronger. When I have had the opportunity to record my blood pressure, which under other circumstances is quite stable, I have found it to be significantly elevated. After the research paper has been given, relaxation occurs rapidly and, unfortunately, the blood pressure returns rapidly to normal. The migraine headache inevitably occurs three to four hours later.

By means of a careful analysis of the relation of certain foods to the subsequent development of migraine headache, I began to eliminate cheeses, bananas, and red wines from the diet. Recently, I discovered a report of foods high in tyramine content and was not entirely surprised to find these foods included.

Chocolate is another substance known to be related to migraine headaches but the substance responsible has not been determined. When I was a child, photic stimuli appeared to result in migraine headache to a greater degree than foods. The most severe headaches seemed to be related to days spent swimming or fishing where the glare of the sun on the water seemed to result in a severe headache. Through experience I found that the use of polaroid sunglasses diminished the likelihood of a migraine occurring. Long periods spent watching movies or television could also result in migraine. The greater the degree of flickering of the movie, the more likely I was to get a migraine. Flickering was especially apparent in older movies or on certain television channels where reception was poor. My only solution to these difficulties was to limit the time spent in watching movies and television and to avoid older films and television stations with poor reception.

Nausea is an integral component of the migraine headache. However, I am not certain that it is directly related to the headache in all instances. Many of the medications taken by individuals with migraine can result in nausea by themselves. Nevertheless, severe migraine in the absence of medication is frequently associated with nausea and vomiting. Immediately following the vomiting the headache may become momentarily more severe but in most instances individuals fall asleep and awaken without any symptoms. I have found that in my case the full course of the migraine syndrome, prodrome, pain, nausea, and vomiting is experienced only rarely and unpredictably.

Before discussing the treatment of migraine, a brief outline of the possible mechanisms of migraine production seems warranted. I have learned that the majority of migraine headaches can be prevented by the utilization of minimal amounts of medication when given at the appropriate time.

In the individual genetically predisposed to migraine, a pharmacologic or psychologic event may serve as the trigger. Either of these stimuli can result in increased secretion of serotonin and other vasoactive amines with resultant vasoconstriction. The pharmacologic stimulus might be a drug such as reserpine or a food containing substances capable of causing serotonin release. The psychologic stimulus might be an acute event or a chronic situation. During the vasoconstrictive phase, the prodrome symptoms appear. As serotinin levels fall, vasodilatation occurs and the headache begins. If the initiating agent is a food or drug, then the vasodilatation occurs several hours after the substance has been taken. If the initiating agent is psychological the headache occurs after relaxation.

An understanding of this sequence and the various inciting agents has helped immensely in treating myself and others with migraine headaches. First, the patient must have an understanding of the migraine personality. In this way he can frequently avoid situations or positions which have the potential of creating continuous psychological disturbances.

Since relaxation frequently seems to result in migraine, I manage to keep myself occupied even on weekends or vacations. Simply setting the alarm at the usual weekday time rather than sleeping late is quite helpful. I noted a decrease in "weekend" migraine when we had our second child who was an early riser. This meant that I had no opportunity to sleep late.

A list of foods known to be related to production of migraine can be given to the patient. As mentioned earlier, these include cheeses, certain wines (primarily red), bananas, nuts, chocolates. One need not abstain entirely but occasionally even moderate amounts will result in intense headache. If I do indulge, I find that an ergotamine tablet at bedtime will usually prevent the migraine.

It is more difficult to abort the migraine when it has its origin in psychologic events unless the individual is very much aware of the stressful situation. I find that medication must be taken sooner and for longer periods of time. I am not, however, in the habit of taking medication continuously. Methysergide has so many potential complications that I feel uneasy with its continuous use. Ergotamine also has risks of toxicity when used continuously. The most effective method of prevention for me and my patients is to cause an awareness of triggering events and prodromal symptoms and suggest taking ergotamine only during these periods. The total amount of medication used with this method appears to be far less and the risk of developing ergotism minimal. One must remember that it is only in the prodromal or vasodilatation phase that the migraine headache can be aborted.

In one of the personal accounts in the literature, a psychiatrist with migraine reported on his own experience. Using various tranquillizing agents to reduce the frequency of migraine, he found chlordiazepoxide to be successful. Drowsiness, however, is an unpleasant side effect of many tranquillizers and may be a greater problem for those with the compulsive migraine personality than for other individuals. Nevertheless, tranquillizers especially monamine oxidase inhibitors, may be useful for the individual who is unable to modify environmental circumstances,

Once the headache is present only analgesics are effective. I do not feel that the use of vasoconstricting agents is warranted during this phase of the syndrome. With mild pain, the more potent non-narcotic analgesics can be used effectively, but with severe headache narcotic agents must be used. The more severe the migraine, the more likely is it that nausea and vomiting will be present. In this phase advice given in a 19th century textbook of neurology still seems appropriate. "The patient should be placed in a quiet and darkened room and allowed to sleep." In the very severe attacks, when no oral medication can be retained, intramuscular treatment must be used. I usually utilize an anti-emetic with sedative effects which permits sound sleep for at least six hours.

Local pressure over blood vessels has been found to be an extremely effective way of temporarily eliminating the pain of migraine. I frequently use this manoeuvre to diagnose migraine. The superficial vessels on the affected side can be palpated under conditions of extreme vasodilatation and are firm with pulsations greater on the affected side. A migraine located near the anterior-superior portion of the head can be reduced by pressing on the temporal artery. Retro-orbital or deep pain can be suppressed by pressing on the internal carotid artery, performed with caution. I knew of a neurosurgeon plagued with severe migraine who wore a tourniquet around his head compressing the temporal arteries during the entire operative period. When the operation was over he would remove the tourniquet and have his headache in privacy.

Much is to be learned about migraine. Genetic factors are present but not completely understood. I think that recent evidence suggests that a biochemical defect is involved in the migraine syndrome. I would place migraine, therefore, in the category of inherited inborn errors of metabolism. Research in this area should be extremely valuable and productive. I am hopeful that it will lead to a delineation of the specific agents which act as trigger mechanisms and a clarification of the interaction of the various vasoactive amines responsible for the production of the symptoms. An effective therapeutic agent could then be developed.

# Chapter XXVIII

# Myocarditis

For a month I had been having occasional fluttery sensations over the heart. Once when this happened I felt my pulse, and it was irregular. I did not take much notice of this, nor of swelling of the ankles. Then one afternoon the "palpitations" turned into a catastrophic experience. My heart began beating violently and rapidly. I felt faint, and as though I were dying. The doctor was called, and I was sent into hospital. By the time I got there my heart had settled down, apart from frequent ectopic beats. I felt shivery and could not stop my teeth chattering. There was a tight feeling in the chest, but not a pain. When trying to sort out the history I realised that the palpitations had only started after a bad cold. The symptoms of this were a very sore throat, a running nose, loss of voice and pyrexia. This had only lasted a few days.

Four days before admission to hospital I had a strenuous twenty four hours. This may or may not have been relevant. After driving three hundred miles I got home to find the horses had broken out from the stable. I chased round after them in the dark and rain without success. The next morning I got up early to find them, and succeeded in tracking them down but could not catch them. So I ran home for a bucket of oats, ran back, caught the horses, and led them home. All this was done at top speed, as I had to be in court thirty miles away by ten o'clock.

The next month was spent in hospital feeling very well indeed. There were one or two attacks of irregular pulse which soon passed off. A month at home followed. At first I was taking propranolol. This perhaps was a mistake, as I was already hypotensive, with a systolic pressure around 90 mm. Hg. I felt more and more tired, and ectopic beats got more frequent, several a minute. So the propranolol was stopped, and the effect was like being resurrected from the dead. After a few more days I could go for half an hour's stroll, and I was pronounced fit for work. I felt very doubtful about this myself, but one has one's pride.

I worked at first part-time and then whole time for about three weeks. During this time I got more and more tired. It felt

as if someone was standing on my chest. There were frequent
attacks of irregular pulse or tachycardia, with difficulty in
breathing.

The next six weeks were spent mostly in bed. The attacks of
tachycardia were frequent. They usually lasted about an hour,
and it was hard to breathe while they lasted. The worst attack
lasted three hours. My heart would beat so violently that the
bedclothes heaved up and down, and it felt as if my heart would
burst. I felt generally ill, with no appetite. There were frequent
shivering attacks, after which I felt burning hot. I would wake at
night with nightmares, feeling hot, and my heart pounding.

At the end of this time I saw a cardiologist, and was admitted
to the National Heart Hospital for investigation. Tests showed
that the diagnosis was myocarditis due to Coxsackie B2 virus.
"Time and rest should produce a cure."

After going home I felt much better, and joyfully set about
some gardening. Either I overdid it, or the infection had spontaneous relapses. Once again the attacks of tachycardia started. I
felt tired and nauseous, with a lump in the throat and a weight
on the chest. The end of the garden seemed a long way away.
Insomnia became a problem. One day I had an attack as catastrophic as the original one, and for a few days after this I could not
stand up without feeling faint and giddy.

By now I had been off work for seven months, apart from a
few weeks. The cardiologist suggested that I should begin work
gradually. I started with a few hours a week, and worked up to
full time over four months. The going was very hard at first. I
felt desperately tired, and had a constant ache in the chest. But I
could manage the familiar routine more easily than I could have
gone away for a holiday. Gradually the nausea became less, and
the attacks of tachycardia stopped. For a long time I went to bed
early and avoided engagements in the evening. There was one
late relapse, which seemed to have been brought on by a cold.

After a year I felt ninety per cent fit, and was fully recovered
after eighteen months. Since then there have been a few not too
serious attacks of tachycardia, and on most days I am aware of
small runs of ectopic beats.

Physical signs were present but not conspicuous. Being a
woman doctor, aged fifty when this happened, the symptoms
were not surprisingly labelled "functional" until I saw a top
cardiologist. The electrocardiogram at first showed only low
voltage and ectopic beats. Later there were inverted T waves and
depressed ST segments. Eventually the tracing became normal.
The systolic pressure was about 90 mm Hg during the first

month, later rising to 120 mm. The heart sounds were not normal, so I was told (afterwards!), the left ventricle lagging behind the right. Ankle oedema, a fleeting rash and slight pyrexia only seemed significant in retrospect. Small changes in the blood count did not seem important on a single test. It was only by repetition that slight anaemia, leucopenia and rise in sedimentation rate showed. The titre of antibodies to Coxsackie B2 virus was 1 in 250. This was done at the Virus Reference Laboratory by a good friend, and was not a common investigation at that time. No virus was isolated from the stools.

Rest was the only effective treatment. I slept well until the fifth month. After that I needed sleeping tablets. I soon became tolerant to barbiturates, but did well on two tablets of Mogadon at night. It was difficult to stop these. The successful way proved to be by cutting down the dose by a quarter of a tablet about every five nights.

It was my misfortune to contract an infection that was little known at the time. It was depressing not to be able to get across to doctors how ill I felt, and I was well aware that they thought it was "my age" — "tension", "You'll soon be right — take some tranquillisers". What a relief to be believed by the cardiologist, to be given an organic diagnosis, and to be told not to expect to feel fit for six months!

# Chapter XXIX

# Obstruction of the Small Bowel

Up to the age of 60 I had enjoyed very good health. Soon after qualifying Ivor Back removed my appendix: I had been his dresser and house surgeon. On and off I had suffered with mild duodenal symptoms but they always responded to easing up on the grog and to the free samples of alkalis kindly supplied by the drug firms. I spent 21 years in the Royal Navy and then took over a radiological practice in Victoria. At 51 I had two attacks of severe colic due to a small calculus in the lower end of the left ureter. This eventually passed and I remained well until a year ago when staying up country in a motel I woke at about one in the morning with very severe pain in the epigastrium of a type quite unlike the duodenal ulcer. It was localised to an area which seemed a circle about four inches in diameter just under the skin. It was essentially a raw burning pain with intermittent very severe spasms during which I had to walk about doubled up. Alkalis and milk and biscuits gave no relief. There was no telephone in the room. My neighbours, none of whom I knew, all had their lights out. I didn't know where the manager lived or how to get hold of him. I thought I would get into my car and drive to the local hospital. However it was winter and the windscreen was covered with ice which I felt too ill to clear. So I thought I would just have to die quietly on my own. I vomited a couple of times and my bowels worked twice. After what seemed a very long time I fell asleep but was very soon awakened by my alarm clock, set for 6.30 as I was due in another town 75 miles away at 9 o'clock. The severe pain had gone but I felt very delicate in general and as though I had been kicked in the epigastrium. I remained well for about two weeks until one afternoon in my office at the hospital the severe pain returned. It was just the same as before, severe epigastric pain under the skin feeling as though it was trying to burn its way out. The area was clearly defined; I could have drawn a circle around it, and there were acute spasms during which I could not keep still. My secretary produced the duty medical officer who called the medical superintendent. He thought I had perforated an ulcer. I did not think

so as one is unlikely to perforate an ulcer twice in two weeks
and all the perforations I have seen had board-like rigidity while
I was unable to keep still with the pain. However without
difficulty they persuaded me to have a bed in the hospital and
have an X-ray taken on the way. A wheel-chair was sent for me
but the pain was so severe I was unable to sit in it and had to walk
to the department. This showed no evidence of perforation or
urinary calculi. I was seen by the local surgeon and a physician
who seemed to think I had an acute ulcer. Two shots of pethidine
failed to relieve the pain. However it eased up a few hours later
and the next morning after an E.C.G. (the physician wanting to
make sure I had not had a coronary), and accepting a bottle of
alkaline mixture I returned to my home. I felt a little uneasy in
the epigastrium and it was tender to touch. On the physician's
instructions I lived on a fat-free diet and took his mixture without relief. I had a cholecystogram, my own diagnosis being gall
stone colic in spite of the pain being central, but this showed
a normal biliary tract. I followed this up with a barium meal but
this, apart from a little doubtful scarring of the duodenal cap, was
also normal. My blood chemistry was normal. I was losing weight;
not only were my pants getting too big at the waist but my
friends were remarking on it, and also my bowels were becoming
costive. The physician said the latter was due to his mixture and
changed it to another. In spite of my suggestions that I might have
tabes, a dissecting aneurism, pancreatitis, hypochondria or Crohn's
disease, my medical advisor still kept telling me it was the old
ulcer. The fat-free diet was causing trouble in the home and I
gave up the mixture as it was not doing any good. The nasty
raw burning feeling was there in the same place nearly all the
time, it was not severe but I was conscious of it. And then, after
about four weeks from the last severe attack, it came on again in
the early morning. Fortunately I was at home and my wife got
the physician to come and see me. He advised hospital via the
X-ray department. This again showed no evidence of perforation.
This time the pain did not let up and, as before, was unaffected
by the pethidine. Two and a half most uncomfortable days later,
during which time I had not been able to keep still because of the
pain, my third visit to the X-ray showed an undoubted small bowel
obstruction with gas and fluid levels all over the place. That night
the surgeon excised a length of intussuscepted terminal ileum containing a benign fibroma as the basic cause of the trouble. I went home
on the eighth day and returned to work after four weeks.

　　And what are my thought in retrospect? Firstly that if a doctor
has to seek outside advice the chances are that he has not got a

simple ordinary condition, otherwise he would have made the diagnosis himself. A follow-through of the barium meal might have produced the answer, but I didn't want to give my time or the radiologist's for this. It is noticeable how with the passing of the years the body toughens: after the removal of a normal, or near normal, appendix in my early twenties I regarded myself as an invalid for several months: after a bowel resection in my sixties I was on my feet within hours and back at work in four weeks.

# Chapter XXX

# Oesophageal Stricture

"Some hae meat and canna eat,
And some wad eat that want it:
But we hae meat and we can eat,
Sae let the Lord be thankit."

Robert Burns

My earliest memories are all of hospitals. Vague recollections of sitting pallidly in the eerie light from an U.V. lamp or of being pushed through seemingly endless corridors in a gargantuan pram are dim in comparison with a vivid picture of a large, white-enamel jug suspended high above my head. From the jug came two red rubber tubes that disappeared into my chest: I was being given a subcutaneous infusion of fluid because I could not swallow properly.

Dysphagia I must have had, but no distinct recollection of this remains before my teens. As a boy, I was the "sword swallower" of the E.N.T. outpatient department. My mother and I would sit patiently until nearly everyone had gone and then I would be ushered behind screens to have bougies thrust down my gullet. The slightly burning sensation in pharynx, gullet and midriff could be easily assuaged with ice-cream later and was trifling compared to the anguish of my mother as she listened to my gagging from behind the screen. In earlier years she had held me on her knees while the bougies were passed.

Occasionally an anaesthetic would be necessary before the bougies could be passed. Eventually the gauze mask held little terror for me, but the terrible, kaleidoscopic bursting of one's head was always unpleasant, and, so very frequently, was followed by retching. Post-operative care was always a delight — ice-cream in large quantities.

About the age of ten, my oesophageal stricture and I agreed on a symbiosis. I no longer attended the hospital for treatment and my food stuck only occasionally. However my diet was

194

restricted. Whatever I ate I chewed very carefully and meat was most often discarded after chewing rather than swallowing. Salads I avoided. Even with these restrictions minor difficulties arose during meals. Something I had swallowed would stick about the level of my lower sternum and refuse to budge unless forced on by a rapid swallow of water. If this trick worked all was well. If it did not, I was in grave danger of regurgitating the water in an embarrassingly precipitate way. At home, I generally left the table to swallow the water, but, away from home, the whole procedure was so embarrassing that I avoided dinners and other social occasions. Rarely the obstruction could not immediately be relieved and once an unusually obstinate green pea stuck fast for three days. At the end of this period I was curiously light headed and nervy, probably more from an emotional overlay than from lack of food.

My growth was not impaired and by the age of sixteen I was well over six feet tall though slimly built. Many remedies had been recommended by family friends, but none worked. I even took Lugol's iodine for a few weeks without any effect on my swallowing or on my thyroid. At eighteen, I entered university to study Medicine. Debates and gaudies were my delight, but dinners and dances I avoided.

In my twenty-first year, on a Friday in February, just after 6 p.m., I perforated a duodenal ulcer. I had had no previous indigestion, only a few days' malaise for which I had taken the occasional aspirin as I thought I had 'flu. The severe pain in my midriff struck suddenly as I was walking home from a students' meeting. I may have gasped at the time, but, as neither my companion nor I were brilliant conversationalists, I managed to walk about a quarter of a mile to the bus without revealing my distress. Some half an hour later, at home, I could only lie rigid in a cold sweat while first the general practitioner and then the surgeon murmured wisely over me. No time was wasted and at 10.30 p.m. I abandoned myself gladly to the oblivion of pentothal. The post-operative period passed quickly and easily and, exactly two weeks later, I went to another Friday night's medical students' lecture where my startled neighbour turned out to be my surgeon. He cursed me softly, but richly, though my rapid return to normal life was taken as a credit to his skill and to the vis medicatrix naturae.

Two days after graduation I went to America. Though the work of a rotating intern was hard and my dysphagia recurrent, I put on weight due to a liberal intake of ice-cream and many nocturnal snacks.

On my return to Britain I faced army service. Though graded P7 due to my history, I was called to Crookham for preliminary training. At the end of my first week, shortly after my first series of inoculations, I again became unwell. Slight coffee-grounds vomiting was followed by intractable hiccoughs. A hiccough is usually regarded as a joke, but on repetition for thirty-six hours, the joke palls. Many devices, including breathing into bags, were unsuccessful. Fortunately for me, an unusually enlightened London trained M.O. came along. He isolated me, put up an oesophageal milk drip and wiped out consciousness with barbiturates. I woke free from hiccoughs and only trivially bothered by a paronychia from army boots. This trifle nearly upset everything as an attempt at surgery under local anaesthesia ended in a general anaesthetic with cyclopropane, which left me vomiting and hiccoughing again. Re-introduction of the milk drip cured me and I was discharged from the army with a diagnosis of achalasia — an interesting observation as my stricture lay some five inches above the diaphragm and the recent upset had almost certainly been due to a peptic oesophagitis.

I became house physician to the Professor of Medicine in my local hospital. The local chef interpreted an ulcer diet as boiled, chicken-drumsticks served without sauce or any other form of garnishing. One of my fellow residents made an excellent omelette which she was willing to exchange for an occasional drumstick. I was so grateful I eventually married her, but not before another episode of ill health. Within three months of starting my residency the dysphagia became steadily worse until even omelettes were difficult to swallow. In desperation I borrowed the oesophageal bougies and dilated my offending stricture myself. This was both unpleasant and foolish, as, later, an E.N.T. specialist, on seeing my barium swallow, refused to pass a bougie.

Luckily I had a sympathetic chief and an excellent radiologist who not only made me swallow barium, but tipped me up when I did so. Actually, tipping up is a very frightening examination when it is done with little warning, in a darkened room fitfully lit only by a fluorescent screen and with the radiologist's leaden fist hard in ones middle. On review of the findings, the senior surgeon said I was "no job for a jobbing surgeon". Leeds was the only place for me.

The lonely train journey to Leeds is wretchedly vivid in my memory. Physically unwell and able only to drink tea, I also had an overwhelming feeling of impending dissolution — angor animae is not solely restricted to angina pectoris. In hospital, I

immediately wrote farewell letters to everyone — letters characterised by bad grammar and their complete lack of taste.

Pre-operatively, I was fed gallons of a rather sickening egg nog
and given a large number of vitamins. Though I knew the site of
the stricture by this time I had no conception of the extent of
the operation I faced. Moreover the operation was never discussed with me. I never had any idea that it would involve a
thoraco-abdominal incision, a partial gastrectomy and a Roux-
en-Y anastomosis — perhaps just as well as I was sufficiently
depressed in my ignorance. A good pre-medication, the hand of
a sympathetic nurse and pentothal removed all worries about
the operation.

The immediate post-operative period was delightfully vague,
though I remember complimenting the houseman on the way
he put up a blood transfusion painlessly despite the large needle.
However, by the third day I felt as if I had been trampled on by
a herd of elephants and cursed a cheery nurse who told me to
"breathe deeply". I have always been rather ashamed of myself
for that. A haemopneumothorax brought breathlessness and fear
of movement, but was rapidly relieved by the slightly unpleasant
pleural tap. By the fifth post-operative day I was out of bed and
walking shakily. On the sixth day I was given a cold, chicken
salad with cucumber which I had never tasted before. The delight
of swallowing without the slightest hold up was incredible. The
colic after the meal was worth it. Eating was grand, but the rather
fatty, foul smelling, loose stool afterwards worried me and I
asked Sister about it. "You've got to expect that now you've
lost your stomach and swallow into your small gut" was the
reply. As a doctor I suppose I should have known this, but a little
advice would not have been out of place from my medical
confreres.

All this is now seventeen years ago during which I have learnt
to live joyfully with "Hubert" — my gurgling anastomosis. My
borborygmi can be obtrusive, but I have found that if I maintain
a stoic indifference it is usually my companion who looks
embarrassed. I now take Pancrex tablets which cut down my
diarrhoea, and I make sure that I take folic acid, some iron and a
monthly injection of B 12. I am still greyhound in build, but
have never lost weight. On occasions I can get a dumping type of
reaction with sweating, discomfort and the jitters. Alcohol
produces a wonderful effect. Because of direct entry into my
jejunum I get an almost immediate flush and exhilaration so that
very quickly I can become the life and soul of the party. I must
slow down there and then and the effect wears off quickly so

that I can watch my companions become "blotto" and shepherd them home if necessary. On very rare occasions I can be laid low with deep seated abdominal pain and aching shoulders, but these bouts are always related to obvious excesses in food and fluid. These minor upsets have not lessened my joy in eating and I am often asked for advice about where to eat. I eat anything and everything, but my capacity is always less than that of my children.

On advice I became a paraclinician so that I could have regular hours. I have never regretted this although I often work long hours and accept as much responsibility as many a clinician. I am happy in my work and never have night calls. Paraclinicians are perhaps a little more sensitive to the feelings of the patients when they have to go into the wards and I for one find much there to distress me. I do believe too, that a period of ill health and a little surgery on oneself makes one more sympathetic and considerate of patients as they lie there, "interesting cases" for some members of the medical profession. Having said this I am fully aware that my survival has been dependent on the scientific skills of many, but curiously enough, my best memories are of the sympathetic art of a few.

# Chapter XXXI

# Osteoarthritis of the Hips

The first time that I was aware that I had peculiar hips was when I began to ski at the age of 30. I was quite unable to snow-plough and found the greatest difficulty in getting my legs into the position of abduction and internal rotation of the hip. The Christie presented no such difficulties. I was 48 when I first began to get pain. The pain was in both hips and in both knees. It came on at varying times, particularly when I drove a motor car and especially a small car with a low seat. When I was 50 I was examining in Manchester and my host noticed that I was limping and persuaded me to have an examination. This revealed gross limitation in movement of both hips, especially the left, and gross osteoarthritis with almost complete loss of joint space in the left hip and reduced joint space on the right. I had hitherto been an ardent tennis player and was now advised to give up, which I did. Gradually my exercise became more and more limited by pain when I walked and after it.

I went to Russia when I was 56 and took a shooting stick for the first time. The advantage of this was that I could walk with it and also sit when there was no ordinary chair. I soon discovered, however, that I could take enough weight on the top of an ordinary stick with a curved handle, and this was much easier to walk with. Standing soon became the most tiresome activity because of pain during and afterwards. Eight years ago, when I was 58, we had some trees felled. I asked for them to be left because I intended to cut them up for firewood. I bought some wedges and a sledge hammer, but unfortunately the smallest sledge hammer that I could get was a 7 lb one. I think that this probably removed the remaining cartilage from my right hip joint, for after that I found it quite impossible to walk with one stick only; I needed two.

From then on my walking became more and more limited until by the time I had two prostheses put in in January and February of this year, I could only walk about 100 yards because of pain. Apart from the incident I have described with the sledge hammer, the decline was quite gradual, but I noticed that if I

injured myself in any way, as by falling over, this usually meant
a sudden decrease in the amount I could walk. I have been
fortunate in that I have had comparatively little pain in bed. I
have usually had it as a result of doing too much or a fall.

I had two McKee prostheses. They did marvellously until I
injured the right one by taking too long and energetic a step up
a steep path when my second operation was five weeks old. This
resulted in my being unable to walk at all without pain. However, I followed my surgeon's instructions and took things very
gently for four months. Since then I have increased my
exercise tolerance and can now walk three miles with two sticks
but without pain. I have no pain at night.

I would guess that in my own case I began with a pair of
vulnerable hips because of very shallow acetabula. I would guess
that I already had some arthritic changes at 30, though apart
from limitation of movement, they were symptomless. By the
time I got medical advice the changes were quite severe. I was
advised to have surgery when I was 56 and refused. I was advised
to have an osteotomy at 58, but found it inconvenient to get
this done. I am very glad that I was able to delay operation until
the extremely satisfactory McKee prothesis became available.

As far as the relief of pain is concerned, aspirin has been the
only drug that I have found useful apart from alcohol. Indo-
methacin did nothing for me. I have, fortunately, never had a
yearning for narcotics. Butazolidin has not been a very satisfactory drug in the people I have known. so I refused to try it.

# Chapter XXXII

# Pancreatitis

February for me has always been the most depressing time of year and the bleak cold days, with their frequent showers of rain, reduce my spirits to their lowest ebb. In addition February has always been the month when I have fallen sick, so perhaps I should not have been surprised when things really went wrong towards the end of February 1969. To cheer up ourselves and also our friends my wife and I planned a dinner party and a colleague, eminent in kidney disease, and his charming Italian wife came along to enliven the proceedings. Six of us sat down to an excellent meal with artichoke soup, roast pheasant and gooseberry fool. Perhaps I was a little indiscreet in eating the fried breadcrumbs, which make such a wonderful accompaniment to most forms of game, with, of course, a little watercress on the side. We had burgundy that night and I was later to recall that it had let me down before; basically I am a claret drinker. We sat talking over coffee until quite late and it would have been a little after midnight when we started heading towards bed having put the second load into the dishwasher.

I felt distinctly dyspeptic as I climbed the stairs, so I made for the bathroom and took a generous dose of Neutradonna in water which has usually stood me in good stead on such occasions. It is a combination of aluminium sodium silicate with some belladonna and I have found it to be a thoroughly satisfactory antacid and relaxant. In bed the pain did not really change and after a while I slept fitfully, repeatedly awakened by this slowly increasing central abdominal pain. It was certainly not the pain that I recall from the early days of the war when I had a duodenal ulcer that would wake me around 2 a.m., nor was it anything like the pain when later I had small bowel obstruction. It was far more severe than either of these and certainly worse than the pain of appendicitis; in brief it was the worst sustained pain I could ever recall. I can best describe it as somebody taking a giant gimlet and boring away somewhere near the middle of the abdomen. The site seemed to be rather far back and quite inaccessible. The odd thing about it was that no matter what position I took up, it remained exactly the same and I know of few abdominal pains that are not relieved in some measure by change of position.

It must have been between three and four in the morning when nausea joined in to make the syndrome more interesting. I placed a bowl by the bed, dreading that something would happen, and then in completely effortless style I had the largest vomit I have ever had in my life. It was what Macdonald Critchley once described as a five course vomit. In the past whenever I have been sick I have felt, like a dog, relieved and full of energy again, but not this time. If anything the pain was worse and so I decided to ask my wife to telephone a friend despite the miserable time in the morning.

It seemed only moments before Dick entered the room and what a comfort it was to have an old friend who is also a surgeon present. We know each other inside out, in every sense of that overused expression, having operated on each other in the past. What better choice could there be? He took one look from the end of the bed and before he even got beside me he murmured the word pancreatitis and in a flash I knew that he was right. What is more my mind worked quickly; I am glad to think that having been a teacher of surgery all my life was not in vain. I remembered exactly where the pethidine was in the house and the next thing I recall is Dick getting a needle into a vein; the relief which followed was unbelievable and virtually instantaneous. I think it is fair to say that from then on I really did not suffer any further pain, only discomfort.

My wife was telephoning in the next room and as usual in London secured an ambulance at once. Two men came tramping up the stairs with a stretcher between them. They were kind, skilful and swift and I take off my hat to our ambulance service which is unequalled anywhere. They had me gently moved and warmly wrapped on that stretcher and somehow down our quite awkward staircase and into the ambulance in next to no time. No doubt the pethidine was working well and my mind was befuddled, but even so it must have been quite a feat and they somehow contrived to give immense confidence. My wife joined me in the ambulance and off we sped. I can remember looking through the windows and seeing the red lights on the traffic signals flash by and then realizing that we must be going straight across them. At some time the siren sounded but I hardly seemed to notice it inside the ambulance and I never associated it with my own visit to hospital.

I was swept into the admissions department and there one of our Australian registrars was waiting and I shall always feel grateful to him too for his neatness and skill in getting me to the ward, a drip up and a nasal intragastric tube down. But of course the only bed in the hospital that night that was free for an emergency happened to be in the Coronary Care Unit, so you can imagine the news that flashed round the hospital next day; inevitably I had been admitted in the night with a coronary thrombosis.

The next three days were uncomfortable, but perfectly tolerable; the pain had disappeared to be replaced by only a dull ache. The bowels simply refused to work and also, oddly enough, the kidneys. I felt sure I ought to be able to pass some water and indeed they put up mannitol in the drip which was beastly stuff which one tasted in the mouth. Also it was quite ineffective in my case in starting the much wanted diuresis. The Department of Chemical Pathology was delighted to report that the serum amylase was well above any recordable limits which they had and so the diagnosis was abundantly clear. Today the treatment of an acute attack of pancreatitis is strictly expectant and conservative. The patient has continuous aspiration of the gastro-intestinal tract until peristalsis returns and fluid and electrolyte balance is maintained by intravenous fluids. As I lay in bed thinking, and there is nothing better than a spell in a hospital bed for thinking, my mind recalled an occasion thirty five years ago, when as a surgical dresser at my teaching hospital, my father had telephoned to say my mother had been admitted in the night to a nursing home and operated upon for acute pancreatitis. I travelled down by train at once to Reading to see her. The surgeon asked to see me and after explaining that he had emptied the gall bladder of many stones and done a cholecystostomy, had gone on to incise the pancreatic capsule and drain the peritoneal cavity. He rated her chances of survival at 50% and my own chief at the hospital considered the prognosis just as gloomily. She recovered splendidly, but what a change has taken place in the diagnosis, treatment and most of all, prognosis of this condition.

As soon as I had passed some urine and even better, a little flatus, I was allowed a drink of water by mouth and it really tasted good. I had a most remarkable yearning at this time for smoked fish in any form. When the medical school's treasurer sent a small pot of caviare my joy was unbounded and it was finished almost as soon as it was opened. I was out of hospital about ten days later still eating smoked fish in any shape and form and continuing to do so for the next month; what is more I still enjoy it. It was considered that alcohol was contra-indicated, but as I usually take a glass of wine with my dinner I made some tentative experiments. I found that a lightly resinated Greek wine, diluted with soda water was absolutely splendid with the sort of diet I had to stick to. I had a diet as fat free as possible and to this day I never take cream or butter, though I do not enquire too closely into the way that food has been prepared.

There have fortunately been no after-effects and no further attacks. I was surprised when I dipped into the literature to find that 50% of people have only one acute attack and no recurrence. It is true that on thinking back I have had a couple of attacks of quite remarkable abdominal colic which were unexplained; perhaps they had something to do with it. Every kind of investigation of the biliary tract, stomach and duodenum has been negative so I suppose only time can show.

# Chapter XXXIII

# Pituitary Cyst

From late adolescence or early manhood I suffered from severe headaches, almost always after playing golf. Over the years the headaches occurred at irregular intervals. In the autumn of 1963, when I was 50, I had a very severe attack with vomiting that lasted for 24 hours. Perhaps there was a sudden enlargement of the cyst with rupture of the roof of the sella turcica.

Soon after I had a motoring and camping holiday in Europe, driving 3000 miles in three weeks. I was continuously exhausted and had to take to my bed. On several occasions previously I brushed the garage doors with my car: I did not then realize that I was losing my peripheral vision.

I was perpetually tired and anorexic and generally ill and was worse after any exertion. I was laid up for 3 or 4 days after mowing the lawn. I had widespread myalgia especially in the extraocular muscles, with pain when moving the eyes, and in the intercostal muscles. I suspected trichiniasis. My joints, especially the interphalangeals, became stiff and there was limitation of rotation and abduction of the shoulders. My sleep was disturbed by restlessness and involuntary movements sufficiently violent to throw off the bed clothes. I had sudden involuntary jerking of the legs suggestive of chorea to a mind groping for a diagnosis. I lost weight and became very pale.

My mental symptoms are difficult to describe in retrospect. I was apathetic and my concentration failed. My thinking became slow and laborious and there was clouding of mental acuity. I lost hair, mainly from the trunk, axillae, pubis and legs and my beard grew less vigorously. My libido disappeared. I became intolerant of cold but suffered from hot flushes suggestive of testicular failure. In the areas of the special senses, I lost auditory acuity and had severe tinnitus. Apart from the garage door incidents there were no optical signs.

Having been labelled a case of virus disease, after about three months rest at home, I took up my duties again in mid-January 1964, still extremely pale and thin, and lacking in stamina. I can remember suffering from excessive perspiration on operating

days, a thing to which I had never been accustomed, but more
seriously I found that I had lost the visual acuity for picking up
small blood vessels and soon my eyes were becoming reddened.
I presume now that this was from continual attempts at accom-
modation trying to achieve a sharp image on the retina. One
morning, in early April, on closing one eye as an experiment, I
found that I was unable to read newsprint and this sent me to an
ophthalmic surgeon for advice. His opinion was that I was suffering
from retrobulbar neuritis, and he ordered a further complete
rest.

It was at this point that on seeking further medical advice, I
was directed along the correct path. It was revealed that X-rays
of the skull showed a large pituitary fossa. Fields of vision were
measured and gave irrefutable evidence of bitemporal hemianopia,
from pituitary compression of the optic nerves, and the diagnosis
was established.

Surgical removal of the pituitary cyst by the transfrontal
route was undertaken. On recovering from the anaesthetic, I
immediately tested my visual acuity for distant vision, and, to
my very great joy, found it sharp and clear, where it had been
blurred and misty. Visual acuity and fields of vision both
recovered completely.

Maintenance therapy has been empirical and it is concluded
that there is about half the pituitary function still present. My
daily requirement of drugs is as follows:-

  Cortisone  25 mgm
  Thyroxine  0.1 mgm
  Fluoxymethisterone  5 mgm

After six years I remain well and able to carry out the normal
routine of general surgery. I do get tired at times, but not unduly
so. I seem to have regained my former mental acuity, such as it
was, hair growth is normal, libido returned and temperature
control seems normal, although I believe that the effects of
chilling would still be prolonged. My warning signal, should I
forget my drugs, is the onset of tinnitus, which I imagine is a
cortisone-lack effect.

May I take this opportunity to express my deep gratitude
for the most incredible surgical expertise, which had me
travelling home on the 10th post-operative day to convalesce
and recover. The diagnosis seemed to be the difficulty, and I
trust that this account may help to expedite this in other
sufferers from the disease, which does not seem to be well
described in standard text-books.

# Chapter XXXIV

# Proctalgia Fugax

The most recent edition of a leading textbook on gastroenterology has six lines only on this subject. The words mean "a fleeting pain in the rectum". It is said to occur most commonly in young adult males and is very common among doctors, but my attacks began when I was 10 and in my practice half the sufferers are young women. Contrary to usual descriptions of the attack, there are, in my experience, three separate types of attack which should be described separately.

The commonest type, is the one usually described in the classical accounts of proctalgia, and tends to take place at night. The patient wakes after increasing restlessness, and if it is not his first attack, knows exactly what is likely to happen. At this stage the pain is not severe, and is cramp-like in character. The penis is erect. There is never any radiation of the pain from the rectal area, and there is no tenderness at all. If the bowels are opened at this time the attack may stop.

The proctalgia worsens over the next few minutes and reaches a peak of lancinating pain. At this stage the patient is usually perspiring freely, groaning, and unable to lie still. From this point the attack will last between 10 and 20 minutes, the pain remaining constant and very severe. Quite suddenly the pain lessens and within a few minutes the sufferer falls asleep with merely a bruised sensation around the rectum. The penile erection subsides at this stage.

The second type of attack starts in the same way, but after the initial onset, the pain does not become worse. It remains at the same intensity, sufficient to keep the patient most uncomfortable, without being unbearable. After a period of up to half an hour the pain disappears. Usually such an abortive attack is followed later that night by another full attack. Sometimes the long period of slight pain is followed immediately by the severe pain; this may be just a variant of the classical form.

The third type of attack also follows the classical pattern, but returns almost at once, to repeat the cycle and produce a second peak of maximum pain only a few minutes after the first full attack. This is obviously the most unpleasant form, as the awaited easing of the pain is thwarted and the patient knows he can expect a further quarter of an hour of extreme pain.

Apart from the third type of attack, more than one attack in a 24 hour period is most unusual. Two or three attacks may take place within a few weeks, particularly if the patient is under some form of prolonged mental stress. Usually there are intervals of several months, possibly a year, between attacks. The frequency of attacks definitely decreases with age. This is also the case with migraine; possibly the emotional maturing of the patient plays some part in this.

As the condition is self-limiting, and as the duration and type of the attack are usually obvious at the start, there is no place for analgesic treatment. Tablets do not produce any appreciable analgesia by the time the pain has abated. More speedy injectable analgesics like pethidine or morphine present obvious problems of dependance. I have never used the newer drugs such as Fortral, in this condition, though they are claimed to be nonaddictive. Inhalation of amyl nitrite and anti-spasmodics are of no value in proctalgia.

Physical methods of treatment give the best results. These methods fall into two groups. The first is some form of anal or rectal dilatation; the passage of a stool is often successful, whereas passing flatus is of no value to me, though some reports suggest that it is. Digital dilatation is aesthetically displeasing, but for doctor sufferers, modern disposable proctoscopes and anal dilators are excellent substitutes particularly if it is not possible to have a bowel action.

The second method involves upward pressure on the perineum and anal region. As most attacks take place at night, the often quoted "sitting astride the edge of the bath", means that the sufferer must leave his warm bed, and add to his discomfort. The easiest manoeuvre that will accomplish the upward pressure is to sit on one's own closed fist, knuckles uppermost and between the ischial tuberosities. This is much the same as estimating the pelvic outlet in a pregnant woman.

Another old remedy is eating or drinking in order to evoke the gastrocolic reflex, but I have found this valueless.

# Chapter XXXV

# Prolapse

It is accepted gynaecological teaching that uterovaginal prolapse can not occur in the absence of a retroversion and that the symptoms are immediate and completely relieved by lying down. They are a sensation of fullness or swelling in the vagina, a dragging discomfort in the lower abdomen and pelvis, a bearing down sensation in the vagina giving a desire to evacuate the vagina, urinary frequency, difficulty in emptying the bladder, stress incontinence, difficulty in emptying the rectum, backache, vaginal discharge and menorrhagia.

I am a married multiparous woman of 31. In my case the dominant presenting symptom of a Grade I uterovaginal prolapse was rectal tenesmus. This was not relieved immediately by lying down but passed off with a night's rest leaving me asymptomatic in the early hours of each day. The only other symptoms present were frequency of micturition and constipation requiring digital evacuation. I did not complain of stress incontinence because I had experienced it intermittently since five years before the birth of my first child. Physical examination revealed a retroverted uterus associated with a moderate cystocele and a small rectocele, and on the understanding that "retroversion alone never produces pressure on the rectum or symptoms related to the lower bowel", (Jeffcoate) it was agreed to insert a Hodge pessary for a therapeutic trial. This however afforded no relief as it could not be satisfactorily retained *in situ* during the routine daily activities and was removed after six weeks.

After the removal of the pessary I noticed that during sexual intercourse the sensation of rectal tenesmus became one of vaginal tenesmus. Rectal tenesmus originally occurred with dramatic suddeness when I strained at stool, but five months later I noticed that towards late afternoon the character of the tenesmus altered from a definite rectal sensation to a vaginal one. This sequence of events reminded me of those in Stage II labour when the foetal head first passed into the upper vagina and produced in me an overwhelming desire to defaecate which later, as the head passed down the vaginal canal, became an overwhelming vaginal desire to bear down. At this time I noticed that I could palpate the cervix uteri at the introitus and my gynecologist then diagnosed a stage II to III uterine prolapse, which he corrected surgically. After the operation I became symptom free and have since experienced only a sensation of rectal tenesmus in association with diarrhoea. The vaginal tenesmus has never recurred.

Before the conception of my first child I wore a vaginal diaphragm as a contraceptive device and the uterus at that time was anteverted. It remained anteverted until after the birth of my second child when the retained placenta was removed by Credé's manoeuvre. After this I found that the body of the uterus lay in line with the axis of the vagina. When the rectal tenesmus occurred I noticed that it was fully retroverted and palpable in the pouch of Douglas.

I would like to suggest that many women who suffer from rectal symptoms in the apparent presence of retroversion only, may in fact have a first degree uterine prolapse which, due either to embarrassment or lack of encouragement, they fail to demonstrate on examination.

# Chapter XXXVI

# Prostatectomy

In my early sixties, occasional nycturia appeared, followed by delay in starting the urinary stream. A urologist diagnosed prostatic enlargement, and confirmed it by intravenous urography. During the following year conditions worsened, with a conspicuous "Chinese restaurant — cinema syndrome". A light dinner with large quantities of tea, succeeded by a three to four hour screen program, found me finally standing before the urinal, waiting for sphincteric relaxation. Lest I aggravate the tension, I forbore to strain. The time had come for action.

My preparations for surgical relief began with a long freighter holiday. Confirmatory urography showed increased prostatic size and the urologist agreed that resection was indicated. He agreed to my several conditions, all of which were met.

First, the use of the suprapubic approach with massive resection; as a pathologist, I am not favourable to endoscopic "revision", so often justifying the prefix, "re". Then, operation either Tuesday, Wednesday or Thursday, thus avoiding the hospital traffic congestion of Monday and of Friday with its relative abandonment of the patient at the weekend. Further, thanks to a now unidentifiable medical article, I would put aside two units of my own blood for use during or after operation. The advantages of this precaution need no elucidation.

In addition, I requested general anaesthesia, even though tracheal intubation would leave a sore throat for several days. I had no desire for operating theatre conversation impinging on a dulled but still receptive sensorium. Last, I rejected the splendour of a room of my own for one with another patient. Despite my preference for privacy, I wanted a potential guardian to summon assistance were I unable to do so. After a telephone call to the hospital, my admission was set for a Monday, and I appeared on the table the following afternoon.

Thirteen days before resection, I gave the first pint of blood, valued at 15.5 grams haemoglobin, and, nine days later, the second, at 14.5. On Sunday, after bathing, I did the major shaving. On arrival at hospital the technician took blood for routine studies and I went up to my room where I found the other bed occupied by a patient recovering from the removal of a vesical papilloma. The pubic barber, appearing late in the evening, showed displeasure at my handiwork, as if it were a sign of distrust in his skill.

Aided by barbiturates, perhaps unnecessarily, I slept well on the two sheepskins I had brought with me. Never during the fortnight in hospital did I experience the discomfort induced by the sheet-covered bed.

Late the next morning, I took a hot bath, a simple prophylactic manoeuvre no one had suggested. To assure good cardio-respiratory stimulation, I walked vigorously in the corridors for an hour before being ordered to bed for the preoperative injections. To my wrist I fastened a tag with instructions: my blood was available,, the electrocardiogram would show right bundle branch block; and would "they" put a small cushion in the small of my back to prevent the ache which so often makes the succeeding days miserable. I told the operating theatre sister of the tag and she handed me a towel. This I folded and placed in position.

That was the last I knew. Early in the evening I came to my senses in my own room. Later, the anaesthetist remarked that I had spoken intelligently and coherently to him in the recovery unit at midafternoon. Of the conversation I had no recollection. An intravenous drip was in position, the indwelling catheter connected to a bedside bottle. I was relatively comfortable until attacked by excruciating cramp-like pain in the suprapubic area which was temporarily relieved by an atropine-analogue. But it recurred again before the next dose was due. This time, morphine gave welcome relief, as it did several times during the remaining hours of the first postoperative day.

My bed was close to a window. The cool night breeze (the temperature often drops thirty degrees from the summer mid-day high), the absence of bed coverings and the sheepskins made me genuinely comfortable between the bouts of pain. Visiting physicians expressed alarm. Wasn't I afraid of catching pneumonia? It was the patient's turn to reassure the physicians.

On Thursday, the drains were removed with less annoyance than stripping adhesive tape from skin. Shortly afterward, with catheter and plastic bag strapped to the thigh, I stepped out of bed, and offered up a prayer of Thanksgiving.

Friday was a day to remember. After a mild laxative, I was prepared to answer should Nature call. She did, not peremptorily, but my response was vigorous, reminiscent of a ship straining at the hawsers as mountainous seas rolled over it. Now

I was excruciatingly aware of the proximity of rectum, bladder neck and prostate. Had I indeed been a ship, when the ordeal was over I would have been awash, every timber under stress. During the next days, the procedure was less and less trying and, by week's end, quite painless.

The tenth postoperative day saw the removal of the indwelling catheter, accomplished with only a twinge. Three days later I was at home, returning to work three weeks from the day I entered hospital. The use of an improvised bedside urinal took care of nocturnal urges. About a month after operation, bacteriostatic drugs were suspended when several urine samples proved sterile. At one urination I passed a fragment which, microscopically, was composed of striated muscle, apparently from the fibres partially ensheathing the prostatic urethra. Libido remained unaltered.

Now, five years later, I have no complaints. Sometimes, in a fit of laughter, I may release a drop or two of urine, but this is a small price to pay both for laughter and relief from the burdens of prostatic hypertrophy. Reviewing my hospital stay, I have no ground for complaint. That I am a male and a physician surely played a role in the attention the nurses paid me and my needs. My professional ego was bolstered by my close estimate, made preoperatively, of the weight of the specimen to be resected. This turned out to be 110 grams, not much above my own prediction of slightly over 100 grams. Of my reserve blood, the first pint was administered during operation, the other went to someone less fortunate. My back never ached and throat soreness from the endotracheal tube disappeared in a few days.

If physicians gave as much attention to prostatectomy in their patients as I gave my own, their patients would do as well.

Chapter XXXVII

# Psoriatic Arthropathy with Thrombosis

In May, 1966, I developed pain over the internal malleolus or the
right tibia. A few days later the right ankle became swollen and I
wondered whether I had arthritis or deep vein thrombosis. X-ray
of the joint showed only thickening of the soft tissues outside
the joint.

My family doctor was in doubt too and prescribed Butazolidin
100 mg t.d.s. The swelling gradually spread up the leg to the
knee after a week, and I still continued at work. At the same time
I noticed a small red lesion on the calf, ¼" – ½" in diameter,
which my doctor considered to be a low grade infection. When I
sought a specialist's opinion he agreed that I had deep vein
thrombosis, possibly with infection, in view of the skin lesion.
Ichthyol paste lint was applied to my leg and covered with elasto-
plast from foot to knee. Although I was not confined to bed, I
rested with my leg up most of the time and occasionally pottered
about outside. Ledermycin was prescribed, 150 mgs. q.d.s., but
this caused photosensitivity with burning of hands and forehead,
and I had to remain indoors.

It was just over two weeks before the swelling subsided, but
there was a little residual oedema over the right external malleolus.
I wore knee length elastic stockings from that time. After a few
days at work, I went to Austria for a holiday in the mountains
as I was told that walking was the best thing for me.

The patch on the leg increased in size and had an easily
removable layer, leaving a red surface beneath. I sought the advice
of a dermatologist and as he noticed a speck of disease in front
of the left leg and some redness around the anus, he diagnosed
psoriasis and advised simple remedies, beginning with sulphur
salicylic acid ointment.

In August, 1966, I noticed pain in the wrists when mowing
the lawn, and a few days later, also when gardening, developed
pain over the inside of the left knee. A friend invited me to go
for a walk and I did a 5-6 mile stint. The next day, pain increased
in the same spot and fluid had developed in the joint, which was

swollen. For this the registrar in the orthopaedic department applied a patellar pad and firm bandage around and below the knee. The next day, the left foot was swollen and I removed the pad and bandage. I thought this was a deep vein thrombosis; the leg became swollen the next day. When seen by the specialist who treated me for the venous thrombosis, I was ordered into hospital immediately with a diagnosis of left femoral vein thrombosis. The wrists were swollen and hurt even when I held a book in my hands. A few varicose veins were now present in the right calf. Investigations were unhelpful: the latex test for rheumatoid arthritis was negative and no L.E. cells were seen. The E.S.R. was 50 mm in the first hour.

I was treated with calcium, aspirin, and later Indocid 20 mg three times a day. Full-length elastic stockings were ordered.

The thrombosis responded to treatment with anticoagulants and the swelling subsided in two days. I was in bed in hospital from 16th August to 6th September, 1966. On the 4th October the fluid in the joint had disappeared, leaving only a little puffiness of the infrapatellar bursa. The E.S.R. had dropped to 26 mm. in one hour and I returned to work a few days later. Whilst fluid persisted walking was uncomfortable. Since this time there has been wasting of the lower end of the thigh muscle above and around the knee joint, but this does not cause any disability.

After returning to work, as Butazolidin did not give any relief, my doctor changed the treatment to Tanderil. I discontinued this after a month because I felt that it was not doing me any good, and the wrists gradually reverted to normal over a period of twelve months. For some time I could not carry heavy things or push open revolving doors with my wrists.

A few skin lesions developed later over the calves and responded to Synalar Cream 10%, applied under an occlusive dressing. Lesions resistant to treatment appeared on the buttocks and I had many scalp lesions with heaps of fine scales. After this, typical lesions appeared on the forearms and elbows with unusually thick hard scabs. All the lesions itched intensely until completely cured. Ultra-violet light treatment got rid of the forearm lesions and some of those on the scalp. Those remaining needed daily applications of Pragmatar ointment for many months. The lesions on the buttocks cleared with the application of Betnovate scalp lotion, 0.1%. The newer coal tar preparations were tried, but made the skin lesions worse.

In 1968 I developed dermatitis of the face and scalp and on this occasion it was diagnosed as seborrhoeic dermatitis; this has

been kept in check with 0.5% hydrocortisone cream for the eyelids, and Betnovate scalp lotion 0.1% for the ears. Pragmatar ointment was satisfactory for the other scalp and face lesions. Since
the episode of August, 1966, the superficial circulation of the
toes has been poor, the skin being cyanosed when warm and
white when cold, and changing slowly over a period of minutes
even in a hot bath.

There has been no further trouble with the thrombosis and no
increase in the few varicose veins in the left calf region and so
there has been no need for special investigations of the legs.

The diagnosis of psoriatic arthropathy seems clear but I find it
difficult to explain the venous thrombosis within the bounds of
a single nosology.

# Chapter XXXVIII

# Salivary Calculus

The most common site for a salivary calculus is within the submandibular gland. The text books state that swelling of the gland before or during meals is pathognomonic of this condition and if some lemon juice is given to taste, the saliva is alleged to be seen pouring forth on the non-affected side, whereas little, if any, is ejected on the side of the swelling.

The symptoms of my salivary calculus were totally different. I had repeated sore throats which responded to gargling with two aspirins dissolved in half a glass of water and to every tablet, lozenge or sucret I could find in my old tuck-box where I keep my "free samples" under lock and key.

I had no swelling of a gland whatsoever: I was sure of that because there was quite a lot of mumps around and as I had not had this disease, I was quite wary.

As I often ran out of sore throat tablets, I used to pinch lemon drops from the secret store my wife keeps in the glove-box of the car: this did not cause salivary colic or any sort of discomfort.

One day I discovered a small lump in the side of my neck. I noticed it again about a week afterwards and I was convinced that it was getting bigger.

Being a hypochondriac, I started to worry about it. What was this lump? Slowly, by elimination, I convinced myself that I had a parathyroid adenoma and as I bravely soldiered on I convinced myself that I was suffering from all the clinical manifestations of hypercalcemia, anorexia, weakness, fatigability, difficulty in swallowing, nausea, hypotonicity of the muscles, the lot.

Manfully, I kept this discovery to myself, but next time I was near my old teaching hospital I waylaid the Senior Surgeon who very kindly listened to the history of my condition, examined me in Casualty, filled out an X-ray form and told me to fix it up with his Registrar when I wanted to come in. I read his note — "submandibular calculus".

Waiting for the X-ray, I was hoping he was right. Mind you, he was "getting on", he did not take very long to examine me, and after all, I had all the symptoms of hypercalcaemia.

The radiologist let me have a look at the wet-plate: the "Old Man" was again right.

My stay in the hospital was most uneventful. Perhaps I looked a bit hurt when the anaesthetic registrar, before writing up my premedication, asked me whether I was a dope addict, but he made up for it by keeping me supplied with PLAYBOY, MAYFAIR, REX, etc.

I was very grateful to the surgeon because the extirpation of a submandibular salivary gland is a tricky operation and he performed it superbly. An incision is made over the gland, the lower edge is dissected from the platysma, which is incised at a lower level and retracted upwards: in this way the cervical branch of the seventh nerve is protected from injury. The facial artery must of necessity be ligated as it traverses the gland.

I left the hospital with a calculus — about the size of a date stone — in my pocket and with a scar on my neck, long enough to justify the growth of a beard.

There are quite a number of men around who grow beards but apparently very few of them have them trimmed. The shortage of experienced beard trimmers was forcefully brought to my attention one day when I was asked to give a lecture to an ancient learned society in a town in the west of England. The trouble with ancient learned societies is that they meet too often and therefore have a tendency to run out of suitable guest-speakers. This was the only reason I was asked by an old friend to undertake this journey. I looked up the train connections in an out-of-date time table, and managed to arrive at my destination hours before my host expected to pick me up from the station. Having time to kill, I went to the nearest barber shop and had a much needed haircut. When I asked the barber to trim my beard as well, he hesitated for a moment, and disappeared out of my view to reappear with an old giggling harridan. He informed me that it was "Mum" who "does" the beards.

I had no option. There I was, harnessed to the barber's chair by a surplice which had seen better times, but still was strong enough to prevent me from moving. "Mum" not only suffered from horrible halitosis, but also from Charcot's triad: intention tremor, nystagmus, scanning speech.

When I found myself outside the barber's shop, I was in a state of near hysteria. I ran as far as my shaky limbs would carry me. Leaning against a lamp post I was acutely aware that people looked at me rather strangely. I had to pull myself together. How? I tried to rationalize: if you fall off a horse, the only thing to do is to remount immediately. Therefore I had to go immediately into another barber's shop as otherwise I will develop a rather shaming phobia. Before I could change my mind I spotted another barber's shop down the street. I forced myself into the barber's chair and had my beard shaven off: "Mum" did not leave very much. Whilst on the topic of lectures, since my operation I have to have a glass of water handy if I embark on any lengthy dissertation, as otherwise my mouth dries up.

At the same time I noticed an increase in the formation of tartar around my teeth. As the composition of salivary calculi is mainly phosphates of calcium and magnesium, closely resembling that of tartar, this is very worrying, because the logical conclusion would be that sooner or later I would petrify. Fortunately I discovered that pink gin keeps the activities of my salivary glands within normal limits.

# Chapter XXXIX

# Sarcoidosis

For six months while staying in a lodging house I attributed my symptoms to the quality of the landlady's cooking and to my own imagination. It was purely fortuitous that a recently qualified doctor happened to enquire after my health and as a result had me fully investigated — otherwise I might not tell this tale. I was eighteen years old at the time and a diagnosis of sarcoidosis was made.

As I remember the onset was imperceptible. A general feeling of lethargy and weakness where moderate physical effort proved totally exhausting is how I would best describe the onset. Loss of all "joie de vivre" with increased irritability and sensibility at feeling unwell might be how a close observer would see the onset.

Sweating early on became a prominent symptom. During the day it would occur at any time (sitting or standing, etc.) coming on suddenly on the forehead and face and then the back and chest and usually accompanied by a generalized feeling of weakness necessitating a rest or sit-down. It would last a short time — 5-10 minutes — and then disappear as quickly as it had appeared. Simultaneous night sweats became progressively more severe as time went on. These drenching sweats often necessitated a number of changes of sheets. In fact this feature led me to suspect pneumonia more than once.

Later a continuous feeling of dull heaviness as though a weight were lying on the chest became a prominent feature. Intermittent short stabs of pain occured on inspiration. Dyspnoea was never a feature.

Anorexia and slight loss of weight were present from the beginning but these became quite severe as time went on. Owing to lack of energy I was unable to maintain the riotous flamboyant image of the young medical student and this disturbed me! I still did not believe I was ill, though my lack of enthusiasm for work and play often made me wonder. After I had fallen a number of times whilst exercising and a rash had appeared on my right leg, a young enthusiastic doctor decided fortuitously to have me investigated. Subsequently I was referred to a physician, and sent to hospital, where a diagnosis was made.

An entrenched reluctance to admit illness or seek advice — well classified in the adage "physician heal thyself" — seems to have characterized my attitude at this time. The interpretation of symptoms as normal or abnormal varies individually but even the experienced observer can be baffled by the nuances and fine division between the physiological and pathological expression of a symptom. In all cases of doubt then — a moral — "cheaper a medical opinion or two than an undertaker's estimate"!

I ·developed a non-nodular rash on the medial aspect of the front of the right leg about midway. A red scaly rash appeared on both elbows — and these became covered with scabs. Axillary lymphadenopathy was present. Apart from looking pale and ill nourished, no other signs were apparent.

Initially diagnosis was based on a chest X-ray. While I was in hospital hypercalcaemia with crystalluria developed in the first week. The blood urea rose sharply and I became semi-comatose. At this point some concern was expressed for my welfare. Steroids (10 days after admission) were then begun, the complications warranting their administration. A remarkable improvement ensued and apathy disappeared. Apart from a urinary infection the remainder of recovery was uneventful.

The treatment consisted of bed rest, a low calcium diet, analgesics, antibiotics, alkaline osmotic diuresis and prednisolone. The last was administered for a year, the initial dose of 80 mg a day being reduced gradually to a maintenance dose of 10 mg. It produced enphoria and a cushingoid facies.

I am none the worse for my experience and the better for the insight I gained.

Chapter XL

# Sciatica, Surgery and Sympathy

Four years ago a surgeon removed my L 4/5 disc. Time has dulled my memory of the pain and discomfort which followed operation and my attitude to the procedure has changed accordingly. Three to four years ago I would have said "stay away from surgery"; two years ago I was in two minds; now I would advise operation if I could find a surgeon willing to do it.

As a general practitioner I would like to develop three themes from my experience of this illness. The first is the clinical plight of the patient with a sore back; the second is the problem of the doctor as a patient; and the third is the need for strengthening of the doctor-patient relationship in hospital.

In July 1965 while bowling at cricket I developed a toothache-like pain in the hamstring region of one leg which I assumed was a "pulled" muscle. I did not appreciate the possible significance of a history of more than ten years of intermittent lumbago dating from my middle 'teens. In August 1966 this injury recurred accompanied by one transient episode of paraesthesia across the top of my foot and this time the hamstring pain failed to improve spontaneously. The diagnosis of sciatica was now an obvious favourite and was confirmed by an orthopaedic surgeon in September 1966. He advised limitation of activity and the use of a board in bed. This advice was followed but deterioration was rapid. Within three weeks of receiving it I was unable to walk without limping, unable to drive a car, unable to use a microscope and required constant analgesia. I surrendered reluctantly and was admitted to hospital with lumbar flexion limited to 10° and a positive straight leg raising test at about 5—10° on both sides. Early in November 1966 after two weeks of bed rest without improvement I gladly accepted the suggestion of operative treatment

Both Hodgkin and Fry estimate that the general practitioner with a list of 2,500 patients will see each year some fifty patients suffering from the "acute back". This probably represents a considerable underestimate of the frequency of backache in the community.

Because of the obvious difficulty in assessing disability in an illness which, unless severe, is more subjective than objective, the complaint of backache has become widely associated with, and by some doctors almost equated with, malingering. Accordingly treatment of backache could often be described as, at best, unsympathetic. Knowing this, the average honestly-intentioned patient is rather disinclined to seek advice at a time when sensible precautions could minimise later morbidity. For the patient whose work depends on his physical fitness this may be of serious economic consequence. I realise from my own experience as a patient that I underused the medical advice available to me through which the final acute deterioration leading to surgical treatment might have been prevented. I also realise that had I sought that advice, unless the doctor chosen had himself experienced the uncertain agonies of lumbago without signs, I would probably have been reassured the first time, tolerated the second time, and thereafter labelled "neurotic" if in Social Class 1 or 2, a "moaner" if in Social Class 3 and a "lead-swinger" if in Social Class 4 or 5.

My approach to the treatment of patients with sore back  is based on my personal experience far more than on any teaching I received as a student. Similarly my attitude to patients with sore backs has become both more sympathetic and more positive since my own illness.

Extending my experience as a patient from the particular to the general I believe I have become a more tolerant and understanding doctor. Even so I still find myself opting out of giving constructive advice when confronted with problems of which I have no personal experience.

The lesson is an obvious one which cannot be re-learned too often and probably applies to us all.

At the time of my illness my experience of general practice was limited to part-time and locum work and my approach to medicine was hospital-orientated. It never seriously occurred to me to ask my general practitioner's advice. The opinion of the consultant I visited was based on his assessment — or possibly under-assessment — of a "symptom-illness" unsupported by positive physical signs or significant X-ray changes. In this field of the "symptom-illness" the general practitioner, if a good one, is king. His advice is based on his breadth of experience of early and minor illness which falls outside the day-to-day work of the consultant, who when faced with this type of problem has to extrapolate backwards from hospital experience into unknown

territory. This exercise is not always successful and frequently
the advice given bears little apparent relevance either to the illness in its perspective in community medicine or to the patient
in the setting of his domestic life.

All general practitioners will relate remarkable and often sad
stories of their hospital colleagues who have treated themselves
and their own families or have gone straight for consultant
advice when the true expert in the field might have saved much
morbidity, often physical and almost always psychological. The
experienced general practitioner rarely witholds the "second
opinion" line of care from any patient about whose management
he has doubt and this is particularly true of his medically
qualified patient. Teaching of students must in future emphasize
more clearly the specific part which the general practitioner
plays in the treatment of illness and how his skill contributes to
good medical care particularly when illness is minor or in its early
stage.

Two weeks of my spell as an in-patient were spent in the corner
bed of an acute orthopaedic ward and for a further two weeks I
was in the side room of a neurosurgical ward. Although it may
seem niggling to complain about small things, I feel I must again
raise two traditional subjects of complaint by patients. One is
the purgation ritual and the other is the relief of post-operative
pain.

The Sister of my first ward was of the old style. A daily
"cross" on the chart was obligatory and, for those failing to
comply with "normality", a frightening programme of increasing
medication was initiated leading to diarrhoea, colic and exhaustion. The technique of the bed pan is far from straightforward
and no doctor who has tried it could for long believe his
"coronary" patients or "hypertensives" or for that matter "acute
discs" are in any way benefited by refusal to allow the use of a
commode. Yet this still happens in many wards. In the second
ward, not once was I asked if my bowels had moved. This
approach is not ideal either but is an improvement on the first.
The happy medium obviously lies at a non-authoritarian common-
sense point between the two extremes. I wonder for how many
patients this aspect of hospital life has made a disproportionately
large and unfavourable impression on the psyche?

The second complaint of inadequate post-operative analgesia is
common, and one to which I must add. After a major operating
list the nurses — but not necessarily the doctors — are over-worked
attending to possibly urgent matters and, because there is rarely

an invitation to complain of pain, most patients suffer in silence. I myself recall no sedation in my first four post-operative days other than two paracetamol tablets on the first night; by the fifth day I, and perhaps also the nurses, were badly needing some respite and I was given the local "jungle-juice" cocktail (aspirin, pethidine and cocaine — I believe) to "give everyone some peace". I slept in a beautiful twilight world for twenty-four glorious pain-free hours. It was like the relief experienced when a teething baby stops crying and goes to sleep. Fortunately, memory of the intensity and nature of pain does not last long and this perhaps contributes to the perpetuation of the problem.

Before discussing briefly and more specifically the importance of the doctor-patient relationship I feel I must record two important positive contributions which my experience taught me. One is the luxury of feeling clean; daily bed-bathing is a wonderful tonic, and, for the ill at home, provision of help to bed-bath is an under-emphasised part of full care. Similarly the physical and mental encouragement from an interested physio-therapist contributed enormously to my convalescence and I no longer share the rather sceptical standpoint held by many doctors to this ancillary service. If the benefits were physical — as some were — then they should be advertised. If they were psychological they are none the less valuable but the reason for their need should be thought about.

This brings me to my last topic, that of the doctor-patient relationship or perhaps more accurately the hospital-patient relationship, for no one really appears to be *your* doctor. Although I knew most of the medical staff quite well, and appreciated that my illness was of benign prognosis, I knew nothing of the nature of the operation to be carried out, of the discomforts to be expected or of the time to be allowed for relief from the symptoms of illness. I was examined in great detail the night before operation by a resident who said he had been told to do this ". . . in case there was anything else", a far from happy thought to sleep on the night before operation and to think over during the three days after operation when the expected instant relief of sciatica did not take place. I received four totally different explanations for this worrying and persistent pain — all on request — one suggesting ischaemia of the nerve, one hyper-aemia of the nerve, another operative trauma, and yet another adhesions; a fifth was also offered, namely that I did not in fact still have pain. The surgeon simply said — from the end of the bed a few hours after operation — that I would be "none the worse for that", a remark open to many interpretations. It may

well be that the doctor when a patient needs additional reassurance and this, as he does not necessarily specialise in the illness
from which he suffers, in very simple terms. I did not get this
and the feeling of fear and loneliness is one I will not forget. I
realise I have done this to some of my patients in the past. I
hope I will not do so again and I equally hope that anyone who
reads this account will re-examine his ability to look after his
own patients *completely* in hospital and in particular, his ability
to answer the unasked question.

To conclude thus would be ungracious. To the immense skill
of the hospital doctors both technically and in the terms of
clinical problem-solving I will always be grateful. For the kindness
of ward and nursing staff no admiration would be too high.

There has developed in hospital medicine and thus in the
teaching of students a tendency to undervalue the roles of general
practice and the general practitioner in the total and continuing
care of patients, whether those with minor or with major illness.
Has this story a lesson? I think it has two. We know that over
the years general practitioners have gladly accepted the teaching
of consultant staff to the benefit of their patients. I think the
patient in hospital would now also benefit if the consultant — in
particular the new super-specialist variant of this distinguished
species — were occasionally to accept the teaching of the general
practitioner on complete and continuing care of illness in the
community. Secondly our patients both in hospital and at home
would benefit if we as doctors were more prepared to evaluate
what we do in the light of honest assessment of the opinions
and feelings of those we treat.

Chapter XLI

# Supraventricular Paroxysmal Tachycardia

I have had supraventricular paroxysmal tachycardia for some
35 years. "Simple" paroxysmal tachycardia, paroxysmal flutter,
and fibrillation have all at one time or another been recorded on
the ECG during an attack. Nowadays most attacks are due to
atrial flutter or fibrillation. Attacks may last from a few seconds
to several weeks. The first was in 1934 and lasted for two and a
half months; it was followed by the removal of a perforated
appendix. Several attacks have lasted over 24 hours. The interval
between them varies from a few hours to several years. Recently,
they have on average been more frequent, but less violent, of
much shorter duration and more manageable. There is no
evidence of underlying cardiac pathology, thyrotoxicosis or
other precipitating disease.

I can distinguish between atrial flutter and fibrillation,
although both rhythms can be wildly irregular. In flutter there
is a fast and vicious pounding in the chest of which one is very
much aware. Atrial fibrillation is quieter and less disturbing both
physically and mentally. These days I can carry out my planned
routine as a doctor during an attack, although at a slower rate
and it is a long time since I have lost time from work because of
the condition. When attacks used to last more than 24 hours
(usually atrial flutter) I sought medical help which sometimes
meant cardioversion. Now with propranolol hydrochloride a
flutter will become a fibrillation, which will later revert to sinus
rhythm.

Heavy or sudden exertion is very likely to start a paroxysm,
but the commonest trigger action is change of position such as
turning over in bed, bending to get into or out of a chair (especially after a meal), or stooping. Excessive fatigue and tension are
both aggravating factors. Alcohol and sympathomimetic drugs
must be avoided. I don't smoke.

A paroxysm may start suddenly from sinus rhythm, for
example when bending over a patient — fierce irregular bumping
in the chest and throat, and off it goes. I periodically get runs of
ectopic beats and sometimes one of these turns into a paroxysmal

227

tachycardia after one of the usual causes, and occasionally without any apparent precipitating factor.

The onset of an attack is accompanied by a feeling of tension. It is not a fear of going into congestive failure as one has faith in the drugs used, in cardioversion if needed, and in the natural history of the condition. The tension is partly because of the uncomfortable feeling in the chest which makes concentration difficult, work an effort and sleep without sedation too readily disturbed. One holds oneself tense in an endeavour to smother this palpitation. There is also the knowledge of an unpleasant interlude ahead of unknown duration which may disrupt one's planned programme and also that of others. Frequent attacks over a short period are damaging to morale, but fortunately the outlook soon brightens when an attack is over.

Some attacks are associated with a considerable diuresis, especially in the first hour or so. The diuresis does not appear to be connected with the type of dysrhythmia, its subsequent duration or the degree of side effects. It seems as though a chemical factor is working out its effect.

The best preventive measure is the avoidance of precipitating causes. Drugs have a more limited effect. I now take propranolol 40 mgm 5 or 6 times a day; on this dosage attacks very seldom start during the night, whereas formerly they mostly occurred during sleep. Attacks by day are somewhat more frequent than they were. Smaller doses of propranolol are not effective. Quinidine sulphate 300 mgm will stop ectopic beats, and an antacid will sometimes have the same effect after a meal. Meprobamate 200 mgm may prevent the onset of ectopic beats before giving a lecture. I have not found digoxin of value so far, either alone or in combination with quinidine.

For the treatment of an attack, physical methods such as breath holding, the Valsalva manoeuvre, carotid stimulation etc. have not been successful; they may slow the heart rate whilst being applied. Eyeball pressure is painful, ineffective and under the hand of the inexpert I fear a dislocated lens. Occasionally by straightening up very quickly indeed at the onset of an irregular rhythm I have felt that an attack has been aborted. These very short bouts may, however, be just runs of ectopic beats.

The treatment of choice now for a paroxysmal supraventricular tachycardia of any cause is to take propranolol 80 mgm and meprobamate 200—400 mgm as soon as possible after the attack begins. Typically, this slows the heart and quietens me within about 20 minutes. Subsequently, some ventricular ectopic beats become superimposed on the basic rhythm, and eventually sinus rhythm takes over. Sometimes a second dose of propranolol 80 mgm is needed about an hour after the first and rarely a third dose two hours later. The largest amount of propranolol that I have used in any 24 hour period that has included an attack is 400 mgm.

Before taking propranolol I used digoxin and quinidine for paroxysmal flutter, and quinidine on its own for attacks of fibrillation. There was never any convincing evidence that this treatment did more than slow the heart rate, or that the subsequent reversion to sinus rhythm was not spontaneous. With propranolol the course of events is now predictable, and an attack is usually over within 4 hours. This is a very great improvement.

Propranolol produces a sinus bradycardia of about 54 beats a minute, and I do not get my normal rise in pulse rate on exertion. In consequence, I am more breathless on exertion than when not taking the drug. There is no bronchospasm, no postural hypotension which could be attributed to propranolol, and nothing to suggest hypoglycaemia. The largest dose of quinidine sulphate which I can comfortably tolerate is 300 mgms three times a day. I have used much higher doses to treat paroxysms and got varying degrees of nausea, diarrhoea, tinnitus and sweating.

The realisation that sinus rhythm has returned suddenly, or to wake from sleep to find a normal heart beat is the calm after the storm; there is also an immediate feeling of fitness again. An attack is followed by a latent period during which it is very difficult to get an ectopic beat, let alone another paroxysmal tachycardia, almost irrespective of the liberties taken.

The pattern of the condition has never remained constant for long, and some attacks will doubtless occur in the future. Running for a bus or going quickly up a hill can be avoided, but it is impossible not to stoop or bend down; I have been caught in attacks so often by variations of these movements. A considerable control over the condition can however, be maintained by one's experience of its peculiarities and by co-ordinating the frequency and dosage of useful drugs.

# Chapter XLII

# Shingles

About 20 years ago I had severe lumbago, diagnosed as a "disc lesion". It has never recurred seriously but occasionally I have had a mild backache, especially after any effort with my spine in flexion. When therefore I got a back-ache I took no notice for a day. That night I began to have a pain in the right loin that felt as though somebody were pushing an apple corer into my right kidney. The pain occurred throughout the night for a few seconds at a time at intervals of a few seconds to several minutes. I began to wonder whether I had a renal calculus or a spinal metastasis and arranged to see a radiologist on the following afternoon. As soon as I removed my clothes the diagnosis became obvious: I had herpes zoster. I then decided to take no further notice of what I regarded as an unpleasant but harmless symptom. I merely painted the skin with collodion.

After a few days this symptom left me and was succeeded by the impression that a platoon of small beetles in red-hot boots was trampling over the right tenth thoracic dermatome. Between these excursions I had a burning pain in this area. If I attempted to brush away the "beetles" I felt as though a blow-lamp had been aimed at my right side. This pain also occurred when my clothes rubbed the skin, so that I had to hold my lower back very stiff and I developed a gait that made my friends ask for the cause and to offer much well-intentioned advice.

The rash developed at first in the expected way, but vesicles did not appear. Painting with collodion merely made me itch, and for this Nupercaine cream was immediately effective. Needless to say it had no effect on the "apple corer" or the "beetles" or the "blow-lamp". After about two weeks the rash began to fade and the more violent symptoms gradually abated, but a constant severe burning pain persisted. It varied in its intensity but was never absent. Firm pressure from a pad I had used for lumbago afforded some relief and I was able to sleep by inserting a small pillow shaped like a figure of eight below my right ribs and lying on this side. I found Mogadon (three tablets) a very effective hypnotic, but either the neuralgia or cramp in the under leg usually woke me at 4 or 5 a.m.

Meanwhile I had tried every analgesic I knew from aspirin to Omnopon. None had the slightest effect on the pain even when doses were increased to the point at which side-effects began to interfere with the efficiency of my work. Whisky however, which I drank only when the day's work had ended, certainly helped me.

The symptoms were not purely local. I suffered from an extreme degree of exhaustion in the evening. When I had been ill for about a month I was sitting in a comfortable chair looking at T.V. and suffering from nothing worse than severe discomfort when I was overcome by a feeling that I could not then and cannot now describe with any adequacy. I could only say to my wife "I feel terribly ill". She turned on the light, gave me one quick look and telephoned to our general practitioner. She said afterwards that I was "deathly pale". I did not lose consciousness but had a strong impression that I was going to die. My memory of subsequent events is vague. I remember my wife and our next-door neighbour (also a doctor) helping me upstairs and undressing me. Soon afterwards I was aware of the two doctors examining me and standing looking puzzled at the end of my bed. Then I went to sleep. The next day, which was a Sunday, I felt glad to stay in bed, although hitherto I had felt much better when up and about because I could not find a comfortable position in bed. On Monday I was back at work and underwent every relevant investigation, each producing a normal result.

I became occasionally very depressed. I don't think that this was like post-influenzal depression because when on an occasional day the pain lessened the depression lifted. This was not altogether a good thing, because a good day was always followed by a bad day and the disappointment was intense.

Other symptoms were noted early in the illness. Extreme constipation was relieved by a Dulcolax suppository on alternate days. I do not understand this, because my bowel habits have always been regular. They became so again when the rash faded. During these same three early weeks I had frequency of micturition, by day but not by night, with a burning pain. My urine was normal. I had an extreme degree of general muscular weakness and I lost seven pounds in weight in the first few weeks. I never had a fever.

I had enough experience of the disease in others to be doubtful about all the numerous treatments my kind friends suggested but out of gratitude I tried them all. I gave myself weekly injections of vitamin B 12 and took daily large doses of vitamin B 1.

I gave myself a nightly treatment with ultra-violet light, which certainly had a relaxing effect. Short-wave diathermy seemed to help for an hour or so, but I suspect that the charming personality of the physiotherapist may have had something to do with this. One kind friend insisted on manipulating my spine and this certainly relieved the secondary muscular spasm. Hot baths afforded great but temporary relief. An eminent neurologist suggested vibro-massage, which my wife gave me morning and evening. It was extremely uncomfortable, but after three weeks it seemed to be doing no good and I abandoned it. I probably did not have treatment often enough because of my full day's work. Others speak well of it. Finally after three months I decided to give up all treatment and hope for the best.

After 13 weeks I began to have an occasional day on which I could not be sure that I was better than yesterday or even last week, but if I looked back about a month I realized that there had been a change for the better. I walked less stiffly and no longer had to restrain a yelp if I had to apply my brakes quickly. It seemed to me that my improvement occurred something like this:-

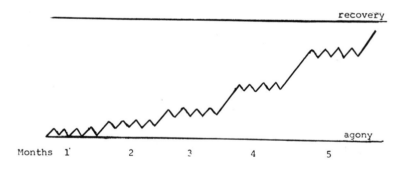

After four months I ceased to have real pain but continued to have severe discomfort, the old burning sensation. It gradually improved in the aforesaid step-wise manner. But I became steadily more tired as the discomfort lessened. Perhaps continuing to work throughout was more than my "constitution" (whatever this may mean) could stand. Although driving (with my back supported by the cage they sell to people with lumbar pain of different causes) no longer hurt, I had to "pull myself together" to face four miles of London traffic in the rush hour and on arrival home almost collapsed into a comfortable chair with a double whisky, my first of the day.

In my fifth month the improvement was quicker. By its end, I was conscious of my 10th thoracic dermatome but not really bothered by it. I had a good deal of itching, relieved by Nupercaine cream. I gave up my pad and my small pillow and slept fairly well without Mogadon. Although I took no more exercise, my muscles improved. Before my illness, although I was 68 and ordinarily take no exercise, I walked over all the Langdale Pikes in a day, slowly but without undue fatigue. At my worst I found it very difficult to walk upstairs and hauled myself up by the banister. In the fifth month I began to walk up naturally again. I remained very easily tired.

After 16 months the hyperaesthesia was still with me but it no longer bothered me. I still lack my previous energy.

Chapter XLIII

# Transverse Myelitis

I was quite well until the 8th of December 1969, when I gradually realised that I had influenza; I was rarely ill, and this, coupled with the fact that I was on holiday, sleeping on a camp bed, and away from the accustomed warmth of a centrally heated hospital, must have made me more than usually slow in realising that I had "got something". I had, in fact, developed supraorbital head-aches; I ached all over; I sat in front of the gas fire for two whole days, and spent the next two in bed.

I was due back on duty on the 15th of December, and duly turned up on the wards, not feeling at all well; it was suggested that I should go to bed, and this I gladly did, with a temperature of 102.8° F.

The next morning, feeling that I really could no longer cope, I presented myself in the nurses sick bay. I was examined, diagnosed as having influenza, and put to bed. I couldn't get warm; blankets were piled on me; I had a heating pad, but it all appeared to make little difference. I ached all over. For the first twenty-four hours, all I did was sleep, and drink plenty of fluids.

The next day, I still had a high temperature, and felt as one does with flu — ill and apathetic. It was not until the evening that I noticed anything amiss, and I think that this was the time that it started. I began to have difficulty in beginning to pass urine; not only this, but the stream was very poor, and the volume small. I was unable to sleep that night, and several times rose from bed and went over to the lavatory, and attempted to pass urine. I was not in any pain, and there was no desire to pass urine — and indeed I could not. Next morning, it was the same, and for the first time, I found that I was having difficulty in standing up-right; my knees were slowly crumpling up under me; I had to make a conscious effort to contract my quadriceps.

By now, I was beginning to feel very uncomfortable. My abdomen was distended, and I still could not pass urine. I turned on the taps in the bathroom, and tried to get into a warm bath, remembering how often I had suggested this to the nurses, when they had reported to me that one of my elderly male surgical

patients was unable to pass urine. I had difficulty getting into
the bath because of my abdominal pain, and because my balance
wasn't very good. The warm bath did not help at all, and when the
pain became very bad, I reluctantly asked the nurses for help.

On the instructions of the R.M.O., I was given an injection of
carbachol; it didn't go in properly and I could feel most of it
trickle down my buttock. It had no effect and so, on my third
day in the ward I was catheterised, and my bladder partially
emptied. I felt awful: I had a temperature of 103, and the nurses
were sponging me with tepid water. I asked them not to, at first,
as I felt so cold, but they told me that it would make me feel
better, and they were right; it did.

I was seen that afternoon by the consultant physician because
of the retention of urine. He noticed that I had a distended
bladder, but there was no other abnormal finding; I had a portable
chest X-ray, and Ampicillin was prescribed. A suppository was
ordered for the constipation that I thought was causing the
trouble. I thought that I had some hyperasthaesia of my feet. We
all laughed at the suggestion of the consultant physician that I
had pes cavus, and my indignant denial. The suppository produced
a small, constipated stool, but no relief of the growing retention
of urine. Later, I was given an injection of carbachol; I noticed
that I felt no pain as the needle went in. I had sufficient response
to the drug to enable me to spend a pain-free night. However,
although I knew that carbachol produced abdominal pain, I was
not prepared for the prostration that I felt, and the copious
salivation. The abdominal pain was not very severe. On the Friday
night I was again catheterised, and when I fell down in the night
during a fruitless attempt to go to the lavatory, I found that I
couldn't get up, and Sister had to be called to help me back. On
the Saturday, further carbachol was ordered, but by late in the
afternoon, in great pain once again, I asked to see the physician
on duty; I felt that I could no longer cope with the "flu", and the
pain and uncertainty of intermittent carbachol.

The emergency physician came and saw me, and for that day
at least, my problems were solved. Having ascertained that I had
indeed acute retention, she ordered an indwelling catheter to be
inserted. I was so grateful for that catheter; I had no thought at
that moment about when it would eventually come out; relief of
pain was all that I wanted. During the examination, the emergency
physician noted that I had a stiff neck, and had equivocal plantar
responses: that same evening I noticed that I couldn't stand, and,
what was more odd, that I had no control over either my feet or
my ankles.

I had a good sleep that night — the last, had I but known it, for about three weeks. But I awoke the next morning, December 21st, quite unable to move my toes, ankles, legs or hips. I remember quite clearly that I didn't feel frightened; neither did I feel particularly inquisitive as to what was wrong with me. I did hope that the paralysis was not going to creep upwards much further, as I didn't want to go on a respirator. I noticed that I could pinch the skin of my thigh, and feel no pain at all; I was aware of the sensation of touch, but not of pain. I traced this anaesthetic area upwards, and defined a border at the level of the manubrium, or thereabouts. My head was stiff; I couldn't lift myself to the sitting position. My "influenza" was considerably better, however, and I read the Sunday papers, lying on my back.

I was quickly examined, and a lumbar puncture was performed. It was quite painless. Then I was seen by the consultant physician who had seen me before. I had indeed a stiff neck; abdominal reflexes were absent, but as I couldn't watch my feet while he was performing the examination, I am not sure of the plantar responses.

By the end of the morning, the result of the lumbar puncture was known; there was a raised lymphocyte count, and a raised protein content to the C.S.F. I was told that the most likely illness was an allergic reaction to influenza, which had affected the blood vessels supplying the spinal cord. The sensory level was T1, and the motor slightly lower; there was also some discrepancy between the two sides. The prognosis was excellent, I was told. Large doses of prednisolone were begun, and I felt confident that I would recover completely. On looking back, I wonder at my lack of concern.

For the next two days, I remained in the same neurological state, without any improvement. I twice had difficulty in breathing, and developed stridor, and cyanosis. On the first occasion I had to be "sucked out". Before this was performed I had no idea how painful it was to be, and sent the physiotherapist flying, with what was practically a reflex movement of both my outstretched arms. I was having difficulty in breathing because of the accumulated bronchial secretions that I couldn't cough up. On the second of these occasions, some friends were with me, and they taught me how to cough, and fixed up a hoist, so that I could drag myself up into the sitting position, to help the coughing. I had no more trouble after this.

Tomograms of my dorsal spine were taken, to rule out the possibility of a space occupying lesion. It was not until several weeks later that I found out, by surreptitiously looking at my X-rays, that there had been a transient scare about a shadow that had been seen on the portable film that had been taken a week earlier. But as far as I know, that was a red herring.

At the end of my second day of paralysis, I was moved to another ward, nearer the respiratory unit, in case I should need the aid of the respirator. This ward was a smaller one. I was given physiotherapy for my chest. Until I was ill, I had had no idea of the nursing care involved in looking after a patient who was unable to look after himself.

From the 3rd day of my paralysis, I began, slowly at first, to recover. It was fascinating to go through the gradual experience of recovering. Recovery was a far slower process than was the on-slaught of the illness. Movement and returning sensation improved side by side. At first, I could move only my big toes; then it spread to include my ankles. Eight days after the paralysis had become apparent, I was able to flex my knees spontaneously and with aid on both sides I was able to stand up. Two days after this I was able to take three steps, with the aid of a walking frame. The next day I was able to take about fifty steps with its aid and a couple of days after that, I could walk the length of the ward, with one person as support.

The return of sensation was not as outwardly dramatic as the return of motor power, but was far more obtrusive, as far as I was concerned. Firstly, I was aware of my feet again and they felt cold, very cold, like ice. Then, at about the same time, I began to wake up after two and a half hours sleep, very uncom-fortable after lying in one position and just waiting for the nurses to turn me, as this was something that I couldn't do myself. Paraesthesiae included a "pins and needles" sensation from hips to toes, day and night for a fortnight; it gradually went away, spreading outwards from the hips towards the toes. My calves felt damp, but they weren't. During the night I felt as though my feet were suspended high in the air, above the level of my head. I felt as if I were lying half way up a mountain, feet towards the summit. Rectal paraesthaesia was even more uncomfortable, and difficult to describe. Briefly, it was a constant feeling of wanting to defaecate. Many times did I ask Sister if I had faecal impaction, for it felt like it.

The most distressing feature of the whole illness, was, however, the failure to return of true bladder function. Initially, I was catheterised, and thus there was no problem. After the catheter had been in for 9 days, it was decided to remove it, to see if there was any return of bladder function. There was not, and after I had been catheterised twice, after developing acute retention, it was decided that I should have thrice daily catheterisation, and that there should be no indwelling catheter. This worked well for 4 days, but bladder function was not improved. Carbachol finally stimulated it into contracting the muscle wall, and relaxing the sphincter. Once the muscular rhythm had been restored, I was aware of the muscle contracting as the bladder contracted, an unusual sensation that persisted for about a week.

However, my bladder was not under my control, but automatically opened itself every two hours or so, if I was recumbent, and more frequently if I was up and walking about. I had a few minutes "warning" only, and there was no voluntary control on my part. As I write this, ten months later, there is no change in this pattern, and it appears that at this late date none can be expected. Bowel control is similarly affected, but this poses very little difficulty, as a regular daily rhythm established itself.

By three weeks after the onset of the paralysis, I was able to walk down the length of the ward several times with no aid, and in four weeks I was able to climb the stairs. By now, I felt quite well, and the only thought in my mind was to leave hospital as soon as possible. I felt frustrated, being confined to my room. In fact I had all the feelings of a normal person who was well, and wanted to be away from hospital. I thought that I should gradually improve in every way, in all systems, but the improvement has not been as great as I had hoped. I can walk quite normally at my pre-illness rate. I can run quite well. I am not a very good dancer and I can no longer jump properly. At night, especially if I have been active a lot in the day, my legs twitch, and the slightest stimulus sends my plantar reflexes upwards.

But it is the lack of bladder sphincter control that is the greatest drawback of all. No longer can I jump up out of my chair, and go dashing out of the house into the road, or go on long shopping expeditions. Going to the theatre continues to be a strain, and something that is better avoided. It is not easy to make new friends, and the easiest way to stay comfortable is to remain within the confines of safety — one's own home. The temptation not to go out is great, and although I think that I cope with the "accidents", when they occur, reasonably well, the frustration that they engender, when they occur, is the worst sensation of all. But this is the only defect that remains, and I am trying to cope with it.

# Chapter XLIV

# Tuberculous Arthritis

Up to the age of 22 years, I had not had any illness other than the usual complaints of childhood. There was no family history of tuberculosis apart from the possible case of an aunt who died in 1889 at the age of 19. The story of her illness together with the vaguely worded death certificate make me think that she may have had pulmonary tuberculosis.

In the early part of 1939, I was 22, and I was in training with the St. Mary's Hospital VIII for the Head of the River. I was rowing on bow-side and there were complaints that I was upsetting the crew by leaning away from my blade. A photograph taken from Hammersmith Bridge during the race shows this clearly. Things cannot have been too bad as we went on to win the United Hospitals VIII's. As so often happened in Hospital crews, examinations began to interfere and we formed a IV in which I had to row stroke-side so that I was now leaning towards my blade. We won the University of London IV's and another race at Richmond before we had to disband. During this time, I was symptom-free.

In late July, I had a long week-end climbing in North Wales. Here for the first time I began to suspect that something was wrong. At the end of the day, there was a disagreeable pain in the groin which radiated down the inside of the thigh. I also found that my left leg was unstable on the rock faces. When put in a testing situation, it was somewhat painful but, most serious it would start to shake. I did not think very much of these matters and did not seek medical advice.

When the war came, I was exempt from call-up as I was only nine months from my finals. In late October I had a motor-cycle crash in which I was thrown and landed on my left hip. From this point onwards, pain became the dominant feature but, as I thought it would get better, I said nothing and went on with my work. At first, the pain only came on when I made a change of position, like getting up from a chair; later it would stop me as I walked about. I think one could call it severe. At this point my friends began to notice that something was wrong (they said I was visibly lame) and they took me to see the R.S.O. at St. Mary's.

After two or three visits, when nothing abnormal was found, I
went again and found that the R.S.O. was away and the Orthopaedic Registrar was doing his list. The examination was
seemingly quite superficial and I was sent for an X-ray and E.S.R.
However, next day I got a call to go and see the late Valentine
Ellis. I had a pretty good idea of the diagnosis and thought I
could get past him. This quiet and reserved man greeted me
effusively and talked away while I undressed and got on the
couch. He asked:- "do you always lie like that". I then saw my
leg, hip flexed and externally rotated. He told me that I would
be admitted at Mary's until he could make arrangements for my
admission to the Royal National Orthopaedic Hospital at
Stanmore and he thought I would be in bed about 22 months.

I went to Stanmore on 10th January, 1940, into a single-
bedded wooden chalet. It was an unusually severe and prolonged
winter. The bed had a thin horsehair mattress on solid wooden
planks. The foot of the bed was raised on 9″ blocks. Skin extension was achieved by lengths of 3″ adhesive plaster from 4″ below
the groin to 2″ above the ankle on the internal and external
aspects of the leg. The left foot rested in a padded L shaped shoe
and the two plasters were connected to a wire which passed over
a pulley to carry the can of lead shot which was the extending
force. My first impressions were the discomfort of the bed, the
easing of pain brought about by traction, and the almost
unbelievable cold. This was the treatment: immobilization and
fresh air. There was nothing else.

About 2 weeks later, I called the night Sister at about 6 a.m. I
felt very ill and had pains in the neck and, I learnt later, a high
fever. The House Surgeon examined me and found that I had
definite neck-stiffness and decided to do a lumbar puncture.
Before he got round to this, I had a perfect rash of German
measles, from which I recovered in a day or two.

18 months passed and the only variation was the climate. The
period had, however one very important side-effect. I learnt to
read. It happened by chance and was perhaps worth the price
paid. One of the Catholic chaplains had access to a first class
private library nearby and he was also able to get me books from
such major libraries as remained open in London. When I left
Stanmore, I was a much more literate person than when I arrived
there.

In July, 1941, I was put into a walking spica and the bed-blocks
and extension were removed. Next day, I had a temperature and
was passing urinary gravel and blood. This extremely unpleasant
episode lasted 48-60 hours and I would guess that I voided about

1 ml of gravel. It was decided to postpone my getting up until my E.S.R. had returned to normal. That day came in the latter part of September. Two nurses got me upright and, with the aid of a walking chair, I took 2 or 3 steps to a short chaise-longue. After about 10 minutes I was put back to bed. This day, so long awaited, seemed to have been a failure and, for the first time, I seriously considered the effects of life-long and painful disability. My thoughts that day turned out to be a wonderful example of over-dramatization, but it is a moment in the history of a long illness which I have since found to be better understood by nurses than by doctors. Convalescence was uneventful and was mainly a time for hard work towards rehabilitation. The hip, was, and remained, pretty painful. With the aid of the physiotherapy department, I got about 30 degrees flexion into an initially rigid knee.

It was decided that I should start work at one of the St. Mary's base hospitals on 6th November. I therefore left Stanmore on 5th feeling lonely for I think I was by now thoroughly hospitalized. I knew that all my contemporaries had gone into the Services and that I should have to make a new set of friends. Also, I should have to fend for myself after nearly two years in which nurses, surely the kindest group of girls ever put together, had protected me from even the most trivial difficulty. It was an unexpected difficulty which first met me; one day I was walking round without a shirt because 2 years of sanatorium life had acclimatized me against the British autumn and next day I was living with people who thought that it was cold and wanted the windows closed and the heat full on.

It was natural that I should gravitate towards the laboratory; this eased the amount of walking to be done and the pathologist seemed to understand my difficulties. After one night in the students' dormitory the medical superintendent moved me into a single side-room on one of the wards for I had not yet solved the problem of dressing unaided. My tenancy of this room also meant that I could go to bed early if the day had been too tiring. After 5 months of this, I was considered fit to manage life in London and I went back to Mary's and qualified in January, 1943. The sector office knew about me and Zachary Cope saw to it that I had a job which would be least demanding on me. However my 6 months as a house surgeon taught me that a long operating list is not easily managed when you are wearing a spica and that night calls are quite a burden when the night sister, who has called you, also has to help you dress to go to her call . . . I have no doubt she would have felt the same, though she never said so.

Professor Fleming was aware of my continuing interest in pathology, especially bacteriology and, in the early summer of 1943, he offered me a post as trainee at the Inoculation Department at St. Mary's and I started there immediately after I had finished my H.S. appointment.

For the next 2 years, I worked at Mary's or at one of the Base Hospitals where I could gain experience. While I was getting increased flexion of the knee, (I now had 90°), the hip was becoming more and more painful and was rotating externally. Finally, I was working in the laboratory attached to Sir Harold Gillies' Plastic Unit at Basingstoke which also had a large military hospital to cope with. The Orthopaedic Units were directed by Valentine Ellis. The Medical Superintendent and Mr. Ellis decided that I should be admitted to the wards on July 22, 1945. On August 20 an extra-articular arthrodesis and osteotomy and an ischio-femoral graft were carried out. I was in a double operating spica for 12 weeks but recovery from the operation was surprisingly quick and uneventful. The spica was taken off about mid-November and once again I began to learn to walk. As before, all efforts were directed at getting as much flexion as possible into the knee.

I started work again at St. Mary's on 1st February, 1946 and continued with physiotherapy to the knee for about 2 months. I disliked being lame and often spent my evenings up in the physiotherapy department practising walking in front of the full-length mirrors. I felt that this policy had paid off when my surgeon demonstrated about 20 adults on whom he had carried out extra-articular arthrodesis of the hip. This was in the summer of 1946 at Alton and I came away feeling that I walked much better than the others. Whether I was right or wrong is really unimportant; it was the effect on my self-esteem which mattered.

In arthrodesis of the hip there are, I think two critical factors: the amount of flexion and the amount of external rotation. If the surgeon gets either one wrong, the patient will have an unsightly "dipping" gait or what is perhaps worse, the leg will not clear the ground in walking and the patient will trip over any trivial obstruction. My surgeon got neither wrong. I think it is not generally realised that when a man is walking along, the amount of clearance between the forward moving foot and the ground is very small and yet the walker adjusts without thought for any irregularity in his path.

About this time, it was realised that the graft had fractured near its centre and the hip became more painful. For a time I considered having another graft put in, this time from the ilium to the femur. In the event I did nothing and, over the years have built up a pretty firm fibrous ankylosis and the position of the hip joint has not changed significantly. It can be painful after a period of strain but I have only had one serious set back. This was in 1966 when I was hurrying downstairs and slipped off the good leg. The left leg was folded under me and the knee was forcibly flexed and the hip ankylosis was strained. I had a haemarthosis of the knee aspirated. The episode has left its mark in that the hip is less stable and the amount of flexion in the knee has been reduced.

In 1962, I had trouble for three months from a calculus stuck in the intramural part of the ureter. It was eventually cured after cystoscopy although the stone was not found. One would like to be able to say either that this was the last piece of the gravel which I had passed in 1941, or that it was a completely unrelated episode but I do not see how there can be any certainty. One can only say that I have had no further symptoms.

In July, 1970 I retired. This was not due to any sudden deterioration in my condition but rather to a combination of three factors: my leg was more troublesome and arthritic changes were beginning to appear in the sacrum and knee; the hospital had increased in size and this meant that I had much more walking; lastly implementation of the policy of zones closed to those not wearing special clothing brought into prominence the fact that dressing was still a problem.

## COMMENT

1. At the start, other people were making comments 9 months before I was fully aware that anything was seriously wrong.

2. Pain was a late symptom but, once it appeared its intensity increased with startling speed. It was the only symptom and I was never aware of night-sweats or even of feeling ill.

3. The extreme loneliness of lying in bed for a long time was eased by the kindness of the nurses and of learning about books. I very much doubt if "light reading" could have been anything like so effective.

4. The intense effort required to become active again after a long period of immobilization. Surrounded by good will and every kind of help, it is still the patient's own ultimate and personal responsibility to get back to a normal life.

5. With a disability such as a stiff hip and knee, there are some things which are frankly impossible. For example, sitting in the dress circle at a theatre. You must avoid such situations, (and they are surprisingly numerous), before you are actually

faced with them, for otherwise your companions will be embarrassed. It was my good fortune that most of my friends were in the hospital service and so I was protected during the time that I was learning how to adapt to these difficulties.

6. When you first come to meet this situation, you feel that you have been hard used but it does not take long to realize that there are very many who have a far more difficult road to travel.